Application of Generative AI in Healthcare Systems

Azadeh Zamanifar • Miad Faezipour
Editors

Application of Generative AI in Healthcare Systems

Springer

Editors
Azadeh Zamanifar
Department of Computer Engineering
Islamic Azad University
Tehran, Iran

Miad Faezipour
School of Engineering Technology,
Electrical and Computer Engineering
Technology
Purdue University
West Lafayette, IN, USA

ISBN 978-3-031-82962-8 ISBN 978-3-031-82963-5 (eBook)
https://doi.org/10.1007/978-3-031-82963-5

This Springer imprint is published by the registered company Springer Nature Switzerland AG
The registered company address is: Gewerbestrasse 11, 6330 Cham, Switzerland

Preface

An incredible amount of money is poured into the field of healthcare every year in the hopes of enhancing results. The healthcare industry is beset by a number of difficulties that lead to failure in avoiding preventable fatalities and subpar outcomes. Lives are tragically lost every year due to a variety of factors, including medical team tiredness, inaccurate patient information registration, imprecise medical imaging, and unequal access to care. Generative AI has immensely influenced various fields, such as education, marketing, art and music, and especially healthcare. AI technologies need a large amount of data to be trained on for various tasks such as disease detection, organ segmentation, planning treatment, and predicting disease growth speed. However, these data cannot be obtained easily for reasons such as disease rarity, clinic regulations, and costly data generation processes. In this case, GenAI utilizes the acquired data to generate new data. The generated data can then be augmented to the dataset to enhance the usage of deep learning and machine learning models. In addition, since the data generated do not expose any patient information and are "artificially created," patient privacy can be maintained effectively.

Furthermore, generative AI can benefit the patient through various approaches. For instance, it can enhance the image qualities negatively affected by radiation reduction, preventing patients from needing to repeat the image-taking process. Also, the generation of one type of image from another more expensive one can help patients save funds. Many tools have been introduced that engage patients more in their treatment process by clarifying and simplifying professional healthcare treatments in a common, understandable language. Generative AI facilitates the administrative process, letting the doctor focus more on the treatment process. It even goes further by helping medical professionals with diagnosis and decision-making, suggesting possible treatment plans according to the patient symptoms.

The chapter "Generative AI in Medical Imaging" explores emerging generative artificial intelligence in medical imaging, a potent way of revolutionizing medical imaging practices. Capable of synthesizing, translating, segmenting, and enhancing images, GenAI holds great promise for accelerating and enhancing many tasks within the field. One major utilization of GenAI in medical imaging is image-to-image translation. Image-to-image translation is the act of converting an initial image into a final image while maintaining specific semantic characteristics. Another application of GenAI within the domain of image-to-image transformation is when synthetic CT images are generated from MRI data. The performance of GANs in generating CT images from MRI has been enhanced by deep learning; however, the outputs often need to be revised due to tissue distribution differences in current methods. Image enhancement is another way that generative models have improved medical imaging. In this realm, super-resolution and denoising techniques are two ways that GenAI models can enhance image quality and increase diagnostic accuracy.

The chapter "Generative AI in Pandemic Prediction" explores utilizing GAN in predicting disease outbreaks, simulating epidemic scenarios, and designing preventive strategies. However, implementing and utilizing generative AI in pandemic prediction faces challenges that affect the accuracy and efficiency of the models. The existing challenges in implementing generative AI in pandemic management and prediction, including ethical issues, data privacy concerns, and the need for stronger and more transparent AI models, are highlighted. Finally, after reviewing previous research, areas needing further investigation are identified, and suggestions for future research are provided. The results of this study can contribute to enhancing prediction accuracy and improving responses to health crises.

The chapter "Application of GenAI in Synthetic Data Generation in Health Care System" explores GenAI models that generate realistic synthetic patient records and images, maintaining patient privacy. These synthetic datasets have the same distributional properties as real healthcare data and give healthcare providers transparent access to information to analyze for research, education, and decision-making without disclosure.

The chapter "Application of GenAI in Clinical Administration Support" reviews GenAI models in healthcare will revolutionize clinical administration and change the face of healthcare interaction in a manner that promises patient care improvement. Intelligentization and automation of clinical documentation make the doctor devote less time to tasks like note-taking and focus on care progress.

Today, patient engagement has become one of the key concepts in improving the quality of healthcare services. The chapter "Application of Generative AI in Patient Engagement" reviews the use of generative AI in this field that can deepen the connection between patients and service providers and provide a personalized treatment experience for each individual. Generative AI can not only enhance patient-doctor interactions but also improve treatment outcomes through more accurate predictions. However, the complexities of human communication and individual differences pose challenges in using generative AI for patient engagement.

Generative artificial intelligence (AI) has significantly impacted drug discovery in recent years by reducing costs and enhancing de novo drug design capabilities. The complexity of drug design, due to the vast number of possible molecules, makes the process challenging. The three key challenges precision, cost reduction, and speeding up the drug design process can be addressed using generative models and AI approaches. Various generative AI (GenAI) methods, including generative adversarial networks (GANs), variational autoencoders (VAEs), diffusion models, flow-based models, and transformer-based models like large language models (LLMs) have all contributed significantly to recent advancements. Recurrent neural networks, including LSTM and GRU architectures, have been applied to sequence-based tasks in drug discovery, while reinforcement learning (RL) techniques have been employed to refine drug development strategies through feedback mechanisms. The chapter "Application of Generative AI in Drug Discovery" introduces these GenAI models and explores their diverse applications in drug research.

Gen AI has the potential to aid in the creation and execution of standardized methods for interpreting genetic information and incorporating personalized medicine into clinical processes. The reliability of healthcare system can be improved. GenAI has significant potential to revolutionize resource optimization in healthcare systems. By utilizing generative AI algorithms, healthcare organizations can improve efficiency, reduce costs, and enhance patient outcomes. The chapter "Application of Generative AI in Resource Optimization in Health Care Systems" explores this subject.

As generative AI (GenAI) technologies such as generative adversarial networks (GANs) and large language models (LLMs) gain prominence, concerns around transparency, accountability, privacy, and bias become increasingly critical. The chapter "Ethics and Regulations in Generative AI" explores how these AI systems, while offering transformative capabilities, complicate classic ethical principles like autonomy, beneficence, and non-maleficence. The privacy risks linked to large-scale data utilization in GenAI, including de-identification limitations and the potential for re-identification, were explored as well.

We would like to thank the contributors of this book for their timely and positive response to the received review comments. Moreover, we acknowledge individuals who have helped us in this project. Last but not least, we thank Springer Publishing Team for their continuous supporting since the beginning stage to the production of this edited volume. We sincerely hope that the chapters of this book can help future research studies not only in academics or engineering domain but also in the healthcare context.

Tehran, Iran — Azadeh Zamanifar
West Lafayette, IN, USA — Miad Faezipour

Contents

Generative AI in Medical Imaging

Azadeh Tabatabaei and Armin ZadZiabari

1 Introduction

Medical imaging is experiencing significant changes due to the widespread implementation of artificial intelligence (AI). To stay up with the ongoing technological advances of our society, including healthcare, professionals need to go beyond and familiarize themselves with machine learning (ML). The hype around AI has both detrimental and advantageous implications for healthcare. In recent years, deep learning (DL) algorithms based on neural networks have significantly contributed to the hype on the role of AI in radiology. These improvements are partially attributed to the accessibility of sophisticated graphics processing units (GPUs), which were initially developed in the gaming industry. We are currently experiencing a progressive but increasingly rapid shift in healthcare from classical skilled practice to a more technological approach.

AI is a broad field that involves the creation of computer systems that can carry out tasks that typically require human intelligence. These tasks include visual perception, speech recognition, decision-making, and language translation. AI systems can be rule-based or data-driven, with the latter category including machine learning and deep learning. ML is a branch of AI that concentrates on developing algorithms that enable computers to acquire knowledge and make predictions through data analysis. Unlike classic programming, where explicit instructions are given, ML algorithms determine patterns and relationships in data to make decisions.

Both authors contributed equally.

A. Tabatabaei (✉) · A. ZadZiabari
Department of Computer Engineering, University of Science and Culture, Tehran, Iran
e-mail: a.tabatabaei@usc.ac.ir; arminzedu@gmail.com; armiz@stu.usc.ac.ir

A. Zamanifar, M. Faezipour (eds.), *Application of Generative AI in Healthcare Systems*, https://doi.org/10.1007/978-3-031-82963-5_1

Common ML algorithms include decision tree (DT), support vector machine (SVM), and k-nearest neighbors (KNN).

A specialized subset of ML known as deep learning employs neural networks with numerous layers (hence the term "deep") to model intricate data patterns. DL algorithms excel in applications like image and speech recognition, as they can acquire hierarchical representations of data. Key approaches in DL include convolutional neural networks (CNNs) for image processing and recurrent neural networks (RNNs) for sequential data. DL models learn to mimic human cognition by constructing a hierarchical model in which more complex ideas are defined in reference to less simple ones.

When it comes to solving the industry's long-standing issues, generative AI (GenAI) could be a game changer. Generative models like generative adversarial networks (GANs) and variational autoencoders (VAEs) have shown great promise in many areas. Since Goodfellow et al. [1] introduced GANs in 2014, there has been a notable improvement with them. Conditional GAN (CGAN) [2] enables data generation for certain conditions or desired qualities, such as synthesizing images of a particular class. Even when there is no matched data, CycleGAN [3] has been shown to be good at image-to-image translation tasks. StackGAN [4] has demonstrated its ability to generate high-resolution images based on textual descriptions, thereby pushing the boundaries of visual realism. When it comes to high-quality images with increasing resolution, Progressive GAN (ProGAN) [5] has produced remarkable results. StyleGAN [6], renowned for its adaptability, generates images encompassing a broad range of styles and distinguishing features.

Medical imaging has become indispensable in modern healthcare, significantly improving the capacity to diagnose, treat, and handle a wide range of medical conditions. From the first use of X-rays to more sophisticated techniques like computed tomography (CT), magnetic resonance imaging (MRI), positron emission tomography (PET), and ultrasound, medical imaging has come a long way. The COVID-19 pandemic made clear how important radiography is in managing infectious diseases. Developing strategies to improve service delivery and effectively address upcoming challenges is essential for ensuring the efficacy of medical imaging in healthcare [7].

AI integration in medical imaging has the potential to transform the field by improving diagnostic accuracy, efficiency, and standardization. DL approaches may improve the precision and effectiveness of analyzing medical images by detecting patterns and anomalies that human eyes might miss. Despite its benefits, the integration of AI raises concerns about data privacy, algorithmic bias, and the need for significant investment in technology and training [8].

2 Milestones in Medical Imaging: From X-Rays to AI Integration

The journey of medical imaging began with Wilhelm Conrad Röntgen's accidental discovery of X-rays in 1895. This breakthrough, which paved the way for non-invasive imaging of internal systems, was the beginning of diagnostic radiology [9].

During the 1970s, the combination of X-ray technology with computer processing led to the development of Computed Tomography (CT) scans. These scans are capable of generating highly detailed cross-sectional images of the body. Specifically in the abdominal region and brain, this innovation substantially improved the capacity to detect and track certain diseases [10]. Magnetic Resonance Imaging (MRI) technology, developed in the 1980s, uses magnetic fields and radio waves to produce accurate images of soft tissues. MRI is a safer alternative for recurrent use than X-rays and CT scans, as it does not employ ionizing radiation. Late in the twentieth century, Positron Emission Tomography (PET) and Single-Photon Emission Computed Tomography (SPECT) provided functional imaging. These modalities are highly beneficial for evaluating metabolic and physiological processes in oncology, cardiology, and neurology [11]. Digital imaging and Picture Archiving and Communication Systems (PACS) in the 1990s transformed how medical images are stored, retrieved, and shared. This digital transformation enhanced the efficiency and accessibility of radiological services [12].

The integration of AI into medical imaging began in earnest in the 2010s. A watershed moment in AI's healthcare history occurred in April 2018 when the FDA authorized the first AI device for autonomous disease screening, specifically for diabetic retinopathy [13]. A comprehensive analysis in 2024 explored 691 FDA-approved artificial intelligence and machine learning (AI/ML) enabled medical devices and highlighted a significant rise in approvals since 2018 and noted the reliance on the 510(k)-clearance pathway for regulatory approval [14].

From the introduction of X-rays to the incorporation of AI, medical imaging has undergone a succession of revolutionary leaps forward that have had far-reaching effects on healthcare. Each technology breakthrough has improved the diagnosis procedure, treatment planning, and patient outcomes. As we move forward, the continuous development and integration of AI, particularly GenAI, are expected to significantly transform the field, offering new opportunities for medical imaging and patient care. The medical imaging historical timeline is visualized in Fig. 1.

3 Digital Image Processing: Enhancing Quality and Extracting Insights

3.1 Digital Image

A digital image is a representation of a two-dimensional image using binary numbers. The object consists of a finite number of elements, each with a particular location and value. These individual units are called pixels. Each pixel's value usually corresponds to the light's intensity at that specific location in the image. Various algorithms can be employed to process digital images, therefore improving their quality or extracting information.

Pixel: The smallest unit of a digital image, representing a single point in the image.

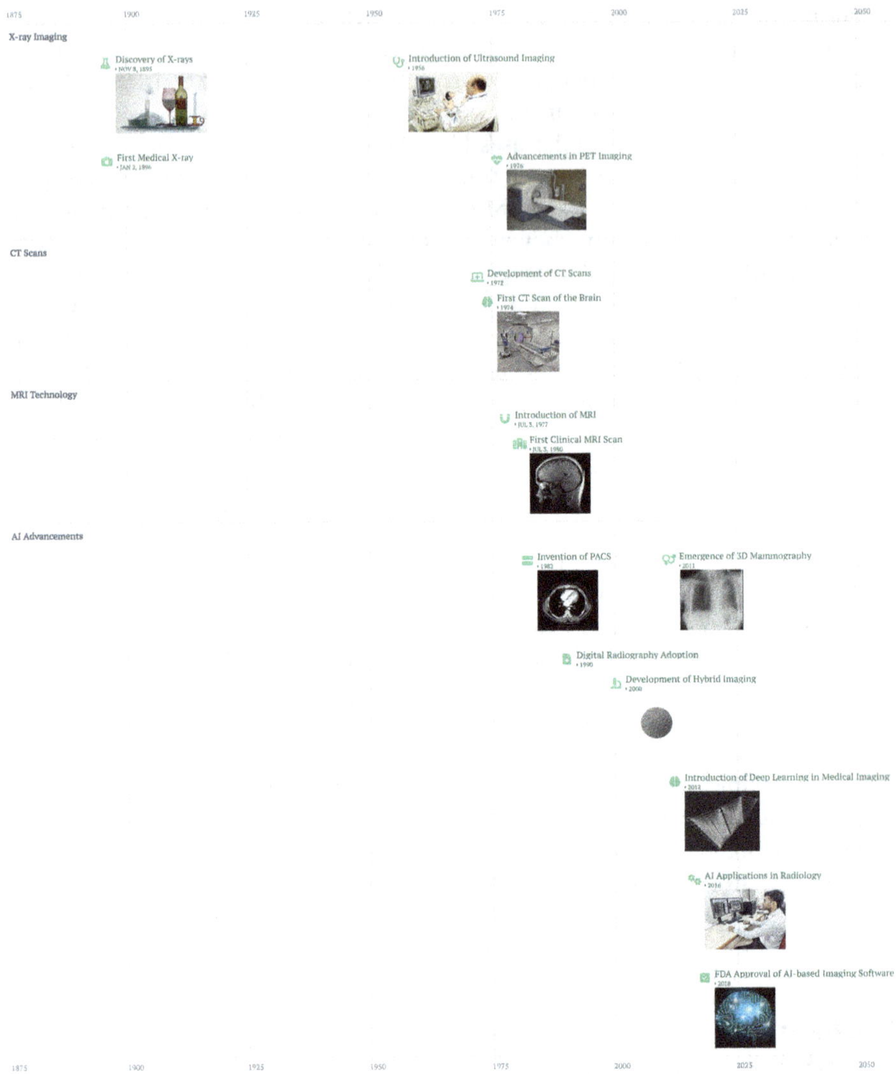

Fig. 1 Timeline of key milestones in Medical Imaging and AI

Resolution: The number of pixels in an image, typically described in terms of width and height (e.g., 1920 × 1080).

Bit Depth: The number of bits used to represent the color of a single pixel. Higher bit depth allows for more colors and finer gradations of color.

Mathematically, a digital image can be represented as a matrix I of size $M \times N$, where each element $I(i, j)$ represents the intensity value at the pixel located at row i and column j.

$$I = \begin{bmatrix} I(1,1) & I(1,2) & \cdots & I(1,N) \\ I(2,1) & I(2,2) & \cdots & I(2,N) \\ \vdots & \vdots & \ddots & \vdots \\ I(M,1) & I(M,2) & \cdots & I(M,N) \end{bmatrix} \quad (1)$$

Here, $I(i, j)$ denotes the intensity value at the pixel located at the *i-th* row and the *j-th* column of the image matrix I. Operations on digital images often involve matrix manipulations and transformations of this matrix I.

3.2 Advanced Techniques in Image Processing

Image processing is a method used to carry out operations on an image to enhance it or extract valuable information. It is a subset of signal processing where the input is an image, such as a photograph or video frame, and the output can be either an image or a set of parameters related to the image. The process typically involves several stages, including image acquisition, preprocessing, segmentation, representation, and recognition.

Image Acquisition: This is the first step, where an image is captured using a sensor (e.g., camera) and converted into a digital form.

Preprocessing: This stage involves enhancing the image by reducing noise, normalizing intensity, and other operations to improve the image quality.

Segmentation: This step divides the image into its constituent parts or objects. Segmentation is essential as it determines the success of the analysis.

Representation and Description: After segmentation, the next step is to represent the segmented image in a form suitable for computer processing. This often involves converting the image into a binary form.

Recognition and Interpretation: The final stage involves recognizing the objects in the image and interpreting the scene.

Mathematically, image processing can involve operations such as convolution, Fourier transforms, and wavelet transforms. Simple examples of convolution filter(kernel) application on a medical image are illustrated in Fig. 2.

Convolution

Convolution is used in filtering operations to detect features within an image. The convolution of an image I with a filter F is given by:

$$(I * F)(x,y) = \sum_{i=-k}^{k} \sum_{j=-k}^{k} I(x-i,y-j)F(i,j) \quad (2)$$

Where:

- $I(x,y)$ is the intensity of the pixel at position (x,y) in the original image.

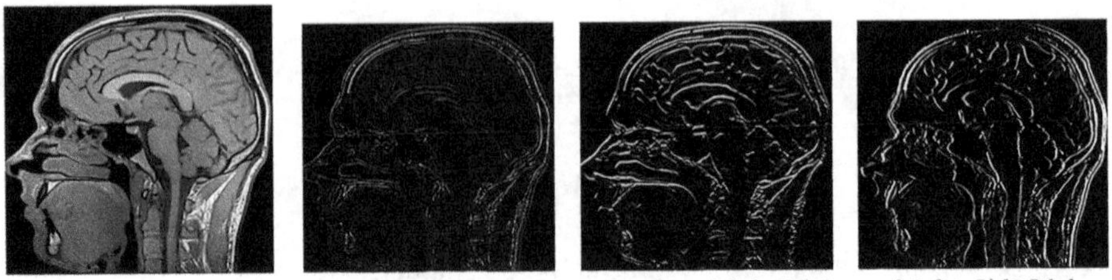

a. Sample b. Edge or Outline c. Superior to Inferior Sobel d. Left to Right Sobel

Fig. 2 Convolution Kernels application on a medical image. A kernel is a small matrix employed in machine learning to extract features, which is a technique to determine the most important portions of an image

- $F(i,j)$ is the value of the filter at position (i,j).
- $(I*F)(x,y)$ is the intensity of the pixel at position (x,y) in the convolved image.
- k determines the size of the filter, with k being the extent of the filter in each direction from its center.

Fourier Transform

Fourier transform of an image $I(x,y)$ converts it from the spatial domain to the frequency domain. It is defined as:

$$\mathcal{F}(u,v) = \sum_{x=0}^{M-1}\sum_{y=0}^{N-1} I(x,y)\, e^{-2\pi i\left(\frac{ux}{M}+\frac{vy}{N}\right)} \tag{3}$$

Where:

- $I(x,y)$ is the intensity value at pixel (x,y) in the spatial domain.
- $F(u,v)$ is the Fourier coefficient at frequency (u,v) in the frequency domain.
- M and N are the dimensions of the image.
- $e^{-2\pi i}$ is the complex exponential function that captures the oscillatory nature of the transform.

The Inverse Fourier Transform is used to convert the image back to the spatial domain:

$$I(x,y) = \frac{1}{MN}\sum_{u=0}^{M-1}\sum_{v=0}^{N-1} \mathcal{F}(u,v)\, e^{-2\pi i\left(\frac{ux}{M}+\frac{vy}{N}\right)} \tag{4}$$

Wavelet Transform

The Discrete Wavelet Transform (DWT) provides a multi-resolution representation of an image. For an image $I(x,y)$, the DWT is performed by applying wavelet filters in both the horizontal and vertical directions. The DWT decomposes the image into four sub-bands at each level of decomposition:

Approximation (LL): Low-pass filtering in both directions.

Horizontal Detail (LH): Low-pass filtering in the vertical direction and high-pass filtering in the horizontal direction.
Vertical Detail (HL): High-pass filtering in the vertical direction and low-pass filtering in the horizontal direction.
Diagonal Detail (HH): High-pass filtering in both directions.

Mathematically, for a wavelet filter ψ and scaling filter ϕ, the decomposition is expressed as:

$$
\begin{aligned}
LL(x,y) &= \sum_m \sum_n I(m,n)\phi(x-m)\phi(y-n) \\
LH(x,y) &= \sum_m \sum_n I(m,n)\phi(x-m)\psi(y-n) \\
HL(x,y) &= \sum_m \sum_n I(m,n)\psi(x-m)\phi(y-n) \\
HH(x,y) &= \sum_m \sum_n I(m,n)\psi(x-m)\psi(y-n)
\end{aligned} \tag{5}
$$

Here:

- ϕ is the scaling function, which captures the low-frequency components (approximation).
- ψ is the wavelet function, which captures the high-frequency components (details).
- *LL, LH, HL, HH* represent the different sub-bands of the wavelet transform.

4 Medical Image Formation

The formation of medical images involves the acquisition of the interaction between energy, such as electromagnetic waves or sound waves, with biological tissues. The characteristics of the energy employed and its interaction with tissues determine the imaging modality, the kind of data obtained, and the image quality.

4.1 Ionizing Radiation Imaging

X-Rays and Computed Tomography (CT) X-ray imaging and CT scans utilize high-energy photons to penetrate tissues. As X-rays pass through the body, they are absorbed at different rates by different tissues, depending on the tissue density. The Beer-Lambert law governs the mathematical basis of X-ray attenuation:

$$I = I_0 \exp(-\mu x) \tag{6}$$

Where I is the transmitted intensity, I_0 is the incident intensity, μ is the linear attenuation coefficient, and x is the thickness of the material. In CT, multiple X-ray images are taken from different perspectives and reconstructed into a 3D image by algorithms such as filtered back projection or iterative reconstruction [15].

Gamma-Ray Imaging (PET and SPECT) Positron Emission Tomography (PET) and Single Photon Emission Computed Tomography (SPECT) are nuclear imaging methods that use gamma rays emitted from radioactive tracers. The distribution of these tracers provides functional information about tissues and organs. Reconstructing PET/SPECT images is mathematically complex, often involving the inversion of Radon transforms and statistical modeling to address the stochastic nature of radioactive decay.

4.2 *Non-Ionizing Radiation Imaging*

Magnetic Resonance Imaging (MRI) MRI employs powerful magnetic fields and radiofrequency pulses to precisely align and control the nuclear spins of hydrogen atoms within the human body. The signals emitted by these nuclei as they return to their equilibrium state are captured and used to construct images. The signal S in MRI is influenced by factors such as proton density, T_1 and T_2 relaxation times, and magnetic field strength B_0:

$$S \propto \rho\left(1-\exp\left(-TR / T_1\right)\right)\exp\left(-TE / T_2\right) \tag{7}$$

Where TR is the repetition time, TE is the echo time, and ρ is the proton density [15].

Ultrasound Imaging Ultrasound utilizes high-frequency sound waves to deliver images. The sound waves are transmitted into the body, and their echoes are recorded as they reflect off different tissues. The image is formed based on the time delay and amplitude of these echoes. The resolution of ultrasound imaging is governed by the wavelength of the sound wave $\lambda = v/f$, where v is the speed of sound in the medium, and f is the frequency of the ultrasound.

5 Image Formats in Medical Imaging

Digital Imaging and Communications in Medicine (DICOM) is the most used format for storing and transmitting medical images. It comprises not just the visual but also metadata such as patient information, imaging parameters, and acquisition settings. The DICOM standard supports a wide range of image modalities, including X-ray, CT, MRI, ultrasound, and nuclear medicine. It is essential for Picture Archiving and Communication Systems (PACS) [16].

Neuroimaging Informatics Technology Initiative (NIfTI) is commonly used in neuroimaging, particularly for MRI data. Unlike DICOM, NIfTI files are typically single shots with a simplified header, making them easier to handle in research environments where large datasets are common. NIfTI supports both 3D and 4D datasets, the latter being essential for functional MRI (fMRI) studies where temporal changes in brain activity are monitored [17].

Analyze is an older format in neuroimaging, used in various imaging research applications, particularly for 3D visualization and analysis. It consists of separate header and image files. The header file contains metadata, while the image file contains raw voxel data [18].

Joint Photographic Experts Group (JPEG) and Tag Image File Format (TIFF) are used for storing individual images, such as in dermatology or ophthalmology, where high-resolution 2D images are sufficient.

Audio Video Interleave (AVI) is used to record surgical procedures, allowing doctors to review, analyze, and educate others based on the recorded content. Dynamic ultrasound imaging, especially Doppler ultrasound, can be recorded in AVI format to capture motion over time.

The Hierarchical Data Format version 5 (HDF5) is increasingly used in large-scale medical imaging research for storing complex data types and large datasets, offering efficient data access.

6 Big Data in Medical Imaging: Storage, and Compression

A single X-ray may comprise a few megabytes, while a full-body CT scan might exceed several gigabytes. The increasing size of medical images presents challenges for storage, retrieval, and analysis. To handle large data sizes, compression methods such as JPEG 2000 and HEVC are employed to decrease file sizes without compromising image quality (see Table 1).

JPEG 2000: Provides lossy compression, suitable for high-resolution images. It is commonly used in DICOM files.

High Efficiency Video Coding (HEVC): Offers more suitable compression efficiency than JPEG 2000, particularly for 3D and series images. It reduces storage requirements and transmission times [19].

With the advent of big data, cloud storage solutions are increasingly being adopted for medical image storage. These platforms offer scalable storage, high availability, and the ability to perform distributed processing on extensive datasets. Nevertheless, the utilization of cloud storage raises concerns about data security, patient privacy, and compliance with regulations such as the Health Insurance Portability and Accountability Act (HIPAA) in the United States.

Table 1 Medical Imaging Modalities Format Comparison

Modality	Image Format	Image Size	Image Dimensions	Storage Needs
X-rays	DICOM, TIFF, JPEG	~5 MB per image	2D, typically 1024 × 1024 to 2048 × 2048 pixels	Low to Moderate: 5–20 MB per study
Computed Tomography (CT)	DICOM	~0.5–10 MB per slice	3D, typically 512 × 512 pixels per slice, 100–300 slices	High: 100 MB to 3 GB per study
Gamma-ray Imaging (PET, SPECT)	DICOM, Analyze, NIfTI	~5–15 MB per slice	3D, typically 128 × 128 to 512 × 512 pixels per slice, 100–150 slices	High: 100 MB to 2 GB per study
Magnetic Resonance Imaging (MRI)	DICOM, NIfTI, Analyze	~1–5 MB per slice	3D, typically 256 × 256 to 512 × 512 pixels per slice, 100–200 slices	High: 200 MB to 6 GB per study
Ultrasound Imaging	DICOM, TIFF, AVI, JPEG	~0.5–5 MB per image	2D or 3D, typically 512 × 512 to 1024 × 1024 pixels	Low to Moderate: 10–100 MB per study
Nuclear Imaging	DICOM, Analyze, NIfTI	~5–15 MB per slice	3D, typically 64 × 64 to 256 × 256 pixels per slice, 50–100 slices	High: 50 MB to 1 GB per study

7 AI: New Frontiers for Diagnostic Innovation

7.1 *Machine Learning Overview*

The advent of the programmable digital computer in the 1940s played a significant role in the advancement of modern AI principles. The field of AI was officially established during the 1956 Dartmouth Conference [20]. AI refers to the process of emulating human intelligence in machines by programming that imitates human cognition and behavior.

Machine learning, a subfield of AI, focuses on software that learns autonomously from accessed data. The learning process involves analyzing observations or data to detect patterns and using this information to make accurate decisions in the future. The main categories of ML algorithms are supervised learning, which uses examples to make inferences or classify fresh data, and unsupervised learning, which discovers patterns and structures in the data without relying on pre-established outputs.

Artificial Neural Networks (ANNs) mimic the functional structure of the human brain by performing complex tasks using a system of interconnected artificial neurons organized in layers. The backpropagation algorithm, an essential component in ANN operations, demonstrates a significant level of fault tolerance, ensuring the system's functionality despite occasional neuronal failures [21].

7.2 *Deep Learning in Medical Imaging*

Deep learning employs multilayered artificial neural networks, allowing DL algorithms to represent and comprehend intricate data patterns effectively. A deep learning system learns not only the mappings of image features to the outputs but also the image features themselves. Some examples of outputs are image categories (in classification), object locations (in detection), and pixel labels (in segmentation). In image analysis, the fundamental architecture of deep learning systems is the convolutional neural network (CNN). A CNN designed for processing images utilizes convolutional layers. These layers compare overlapping rectangular patches of the input image to small weight matrices, known as kernels or filters, that encode features [22].

Self-supervised learning (SSL) has emerged as a powerful paradigm in medical imaging, addressing the challenge of limited annotated data by leveraging large amounts of unlabeled data to learn robust representations. SSL involves creating auxiliary tasks, known as pretext tasks, that do not require manual annotations. These tasks enable models to learn useful features from the data itself. SSL methods can be broadly categorized into predictive, generative, and contrastive approaches [23]. One major challenge is the high global similarity of medical images, which can hamper the performance of instance discrimination methods. Researchers have developed context-aware instance discrimination techniques to capture finer contextual information from medical images [24].

7.3 *Computer Vision Tasks in Medical Imaging*

Computer vision in medical imaging encompasses a variety of tasks aimed at enhancing diagnostic accuracy, treatment planning, and overall patient care (Fig. 3).

Image classification in medical imaging involves categorizing images into predefined classes, such as identifying various tumor kinds or distinguishing between healthy and diseased tissues. Deep models, particularly Convolutional Neural Networks (CNNs), have demonstrated remarkable achievements in this domain. For instance, synergic deep learning models using multiple CNNs simultaneously have achieved state-of-the-art performance in medical image classification tasks [25].

Object detection in medical imaging involves detecting and localizing objects of interest, such as tumors or anatomical structures, within an image. Techniques like the MS Transformer, which uses a self-supervised learning approach and hierarchical transformer model, have been developed to address challenges such as low resolution and high noise in medical images [26]. Additionally, models like SOCR-YOLO have been designed to detect small-scale abnormalities with high accuracy and efficiency [27].

Image segmentation is the process of partitioning an image into meaningful regions, often corresponding to different anatomical structures or pathological

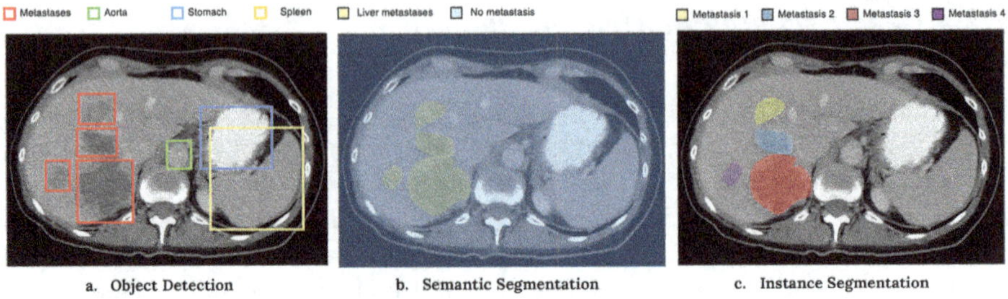

Fig. 3 Computer Vision tasks on axial contrast-enhanced CT scans. (**a**) Object detection identifies lesions, structures, or organs (e.g., liver metastases are in red squares, the aorta is in a green square, the stomach is in a blue square, and the spleen is in a yellow square). (**b**) Semantic segmentation assigns an object category label to each pixel in the image (e.g., all liver metastases are in yellow). (**c**) Instance segmentation assigns individual labels to each pixel in the image (e.g., individual liver metastases are segmented in red, blue, purple, and yellow) [22]

areas. Deep learning-based methods, such as U-Net and fully convolutional networks, have significantly improved segmentation accuracy. Multimodal image analysis using deep convolutional neural networks has shown superior performance in segmenting soft tissue sarcomas from MRI, CT, and PET images [28]. The Segment Anything Model (SAM) has also emerged as a promising solution for medical image segmentation due to its zero-shot capability [29].

Image registration entails the alignment of images from various time points, modalities, or patients to a common coordinate system. This task is essential for tracking disease progression, combining information from multiple imaging modalities, and planning surgical interventions. Techniques such as intensity-based registration and the use of SIFT and SURF algorithms have been employed to improve the accuracy and efficiency of image registration [30].

Image synthesis in medical imaging involves generating new images that are realistic and useful for various applications, such as data augmentation and training of machine learning models. Generative Adversarial Networks (GANs) have been widely used for this purpose, enabling the generation of realistic medical images and corresponding annotations [31]. Recent advancements in diffusion models have also shown promise in generating photorealistic medical images, which can help preserve patient anonymity and enhance data sharing for research [32].

8 Generative Models in Medical Imaging

Generative Artificial Intelligence (GenAI) is rapidly transforming various domains, including healthcare. In the specific context of medical imaging, GenAI refers to a category of algorithms that can generate new data samples from learned distributions of input data. These algorithms are essential for tasks like data augmentation, image reconstruction, denoising, anomaly detection, and facilitating diagnostic

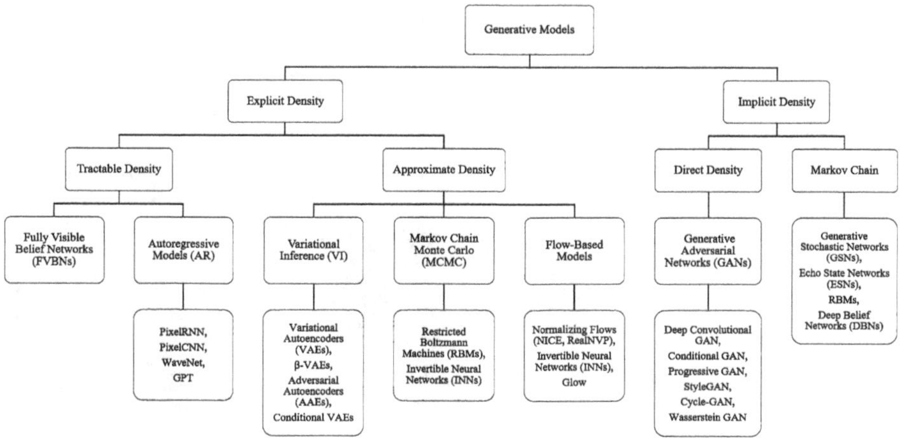

Fig. 4 Generative Models Taxonomy

processes by extending human visual perception. Various types of generative models have been developed, each with a specific set of functionalities. Figure 4 presents a taxonomy of generative models.

Consider the example in Fig. 5, reconstruct areas of anatomical locations in the medical image created by using DALL-E 2. The bordered regions of the original images were removed before providing the remnant images for reconstruction [33]. The model learned the underlying distribution from existing scans and was able to produce a new data that closely resembles the original data, illustrating the power of generative models in creating realistic medical imagery.

The generative models commonly used in medical imaging can be broadly categorized into:

- Autoregressive Models (AR)
- Variational Autoencoders (VAEs)
- Generative Adversarial Networks (GANs)
- Flow-Based Models
- Diffusion Models

8.1 Autoregressive Models (AR)

Autoregressive models generate images one pixel or patch at a time, conditioning each new pixel on the previously generated pixels. **Fully Visible Belief Networks (FVBN)** are a type of autoregressive generative model that explicitly models the joint probability distribution of the data (such as pixels in an image) by decomposing it into a series of conditional probabilities. In this way, the model generates each element (e.g., pixel) by conditioning the previously generated elements, ensuring a

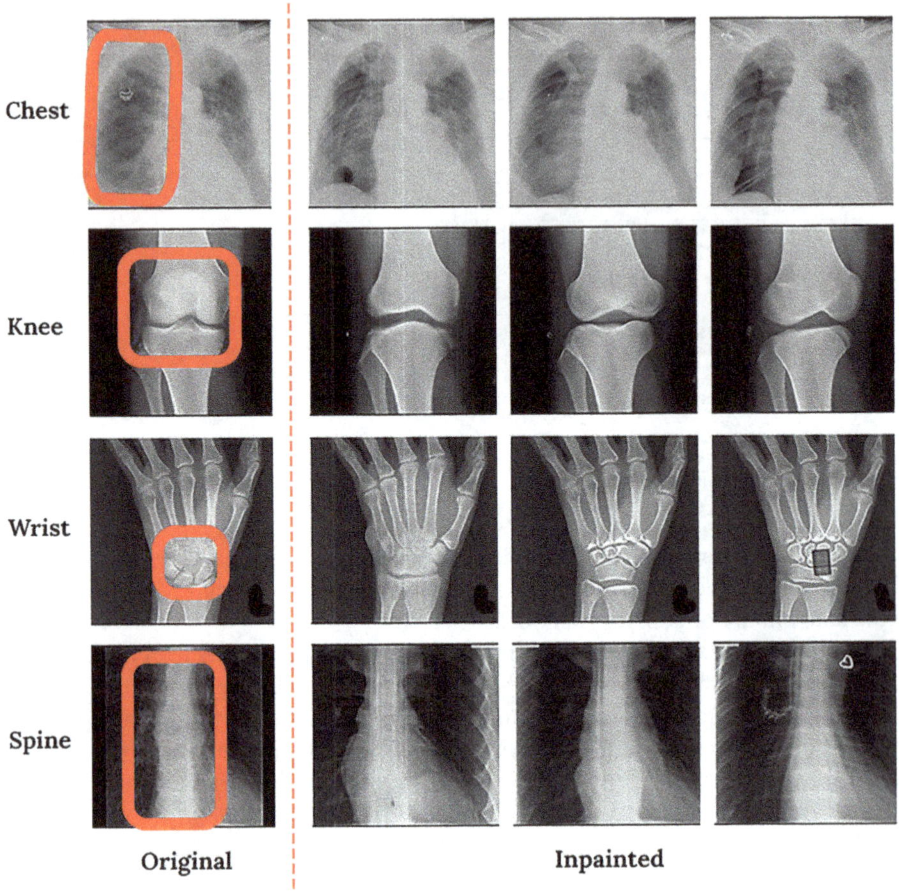

Fig. 5 Reconstructed areas of medical images using DALL-E 2

coherent structure. For a data sample $x = (x_1, x_2, \ldots, x_n)$, where x could be the pixel values of an image, FVBN models the joint probability distribution as:

$$p(x) = p(x_1)\,p(x_2 \mid x_1)\,p(x_3 \mid x_1, x_2)\cdots p(x_n \mid x_1, x_2, \ldots, x_{n-1}) \tag{8}$$

This decomposition of the joint probability is what makes the model "fully visible," meaning that the generation of each new variable (or pixel) is entirely dependent on the previously visible ones. These models are known for their ability to produce high-quality images but are computationally intensive.

PixelRNN and PixelCNN are two well-known autoregressive models used for image generation.

PixelRNN: This model generates images by predicting each pixel sequentially, one after the other, while scanning the image in a raster scan order (left to right, top

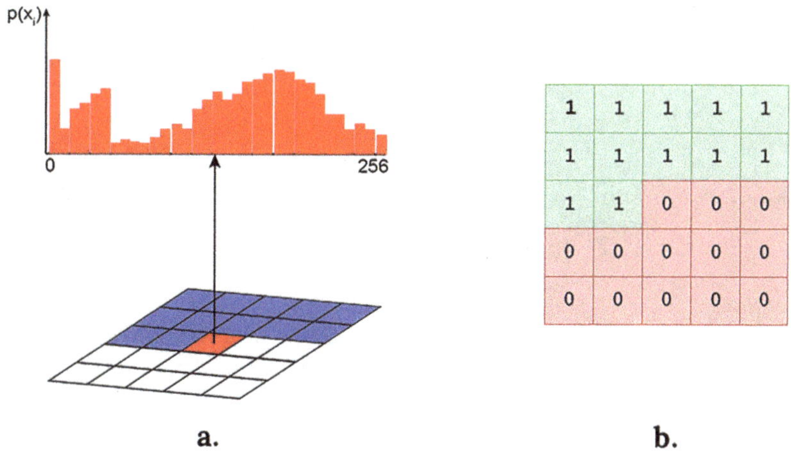

Fig. 6 Illustration of Causal Convolution in the PixelCNN. (**a**) Predicted Probabilities at each pixel, (**b**) Mask Matrices

to bottom). PixelRNN uses recurrent neural networks (LSTM) to model the dependencies between pixels. The RNNs allow the model to maintain a memory of the previously generated pixels, which helps in making informed predictions for the next pixel [34].

PixelCNN: Similar to PixelRNN, PixelCNN also generates images by predicting one pixel at a time. However, instead of using RNNs, PixelCNN uses convolutional neural networks (CNNs) to model the pixel dependencies (see Fig. 6). The convolutional layers allow the model to efficiently capture local dependencies between pixels, making the generation process faster than PixelRNN [35, 36]

Applications and Limitations:

- High-Resolution Image Synthesis: Autoregressive models can generate detailed, high-resolution medical images, although they are slower than other methods.
- Sequential Image Generation: These models are applicable in tasks that require sequential generating.

8.2 Variational Autoencoders (VAEs)

VAEs are probabilistic generative models based on autoencoders, which were introduced by Kingma & Welling in 2013 [37]. One of the main benefits of VAEs in medical image analysis is their ability to learn a lower-dimensional representation of input images. VAEs are composed of an encoder network that maps the input image to a probabilistic latent space modeled by a Gaussian distribution and a decoder network that reconstructs the image from the latent representation. The VAE model consists of an encoder network $q_\theta(z|x)$ that maps the input data x to a latent representation z and a decoder network $p_\theta(x|z)$ that reconstructs the data from the latent space. The VAE objective is to maximize the evidence lower bound (ELBO):

$$ELBO(\theta,\phi;x) = E_{q_\phi(z|x)}\left[\log p_\theta(x|z)\right] - D_{KL}\left(q_\phi(z|x)\|p(z)\right) \tag{9}$$

Where D_{KL} is the Kullback-Leibler divergence between the encoder's distribution $q_\theta(z|x)$ and the prior distribution $p(z)$, often chosen as a standard normal distribution.

Applications
VAEs are used in medical imaging for data augmentation, anomaly detection, and image reconstruction. They help in generating synthetic medical images, which can augment limited datasets, thus improving model training [38]. VAEs are also employed in unsupervised anomaly detection, such as lesion detection, by learning the distribution of normal images and identifying deviations [39].

Limitations VAEs often produce less sharp images compared to other models like GANs. They also face challenges with variance shrinkage, which can affect the accuracy of anomaly detection [40].

Generative AI is revolutionizing disease diagnosis by significantly improving the analysis of medical images such as X-rays, MRIs, and CT scans. By harnessing advanced deep learning algorithms, generative models can synthesize, enhance, and interpret medical images with remarkable accuracy. This enables more precise detection of diseases and assists in identifying early-stage conditions like cancer, cardiovascular diseases, and neurological disorders. Trained on vast datasets, generative AI can uncover subtle patterns that may go unnoticed by the human eye, facilitating quicker diagnoses and more tailored treatment plans. Importantly, this technology offers non-invasive diagnostic alternatives, reducing the need for invasive procedures and contributing to more efficient and accessible healthcare solutions [41, 42].

In the realm of medical image segmentation [43], generative AI has also been utilized to delineate organ boundaries and highlight regions of interest that could indicate underlying conditions, as well as generate radiology reports [44]. This is particularly vital in conditions like cancer, where accuracy in image segmentation directly influences diagnosis and treatment decisions such as biopsies, radiotherapy or surgeries. Specifically, generative models like Generative Adversarial Networks (GANs) and Variational Autoencoders (VAEs) have been highly effective in analyzing CT scans of the lungs. GANs can enhance low-quality images, enabling the detection of minute lung nodules that might signify early-stage cancer [45–47]. VAEs offer probabilistic representations by learning latent features of healthy and cancerous tissues, improving the accuracy of malignancy predictions. These models can even simulate disease progression, helping radiologists differentiate between benign and malignant nodules over time. By accelerating the diagnostic process and reducing false positives, generative AI not only enhances lung cancer diagnosis but also improves patient outcomes through earlier and more precise interventions [41, 44].

8.3 Generative Adversarial Networks (GANs)

GANs, introduced by Goodfellow et al. in 2014, have become one of the most influential models in GenAI.[1] A GAN consists of two neural networks, a generator *G* and a discriminator *D*, which are trained simultaneously [1] and competing against each other. The generator tries to produce realistic synthetic data from a random noise vector *z*, typically sampled from a simple distribution such as a Gaussian. The discriminator, on the other hand, evaluates whether a given sample is real (from the training data) or fake (produced by the generator). The training process is a minimax game, described by the following objective function:

$$\min_G \max_D E_{x \sim p_{data}(x)}\left[logD(x)\right] + E_{z \sim p_z(z)}\left[\log\left(1 - D\left(G(z)\right)\right)\right] \tag{10}$$

Applications

- Data Augmentation: GANs are extensively used for data augmentation in medical imaging to address the scarcity of labeled data, especially in rare disease cases. Techniques like SSA-CycleGAN and SAG-GAN have been developed to generate synthetic images, enhancing the training datasets and improving classification performance [48, 49].
- Image-to-Image Translation: GANs facilitate image-to-image translation tasks such as MRI to CT scan conversion, super-resolution, and denoising. Models like CycleGAN and Pix2Pix are employed for cross-modality synthesis and improving image quality [31, 50].
- Reconstruction from Incomplete Data: GANs are applied to reconstruct high-quality images from incomplete data, such as in compressed sensing MRI (CS-MRI). Techniques like HARA-GAN and DU-GAN enhance image quality and reduce scanning time, improving patient comfort [51, 52].

Limitations GANs face challenges like mode collapse, instability, and the need for large datasets. These issues can affect the quality and reliability of generated images, necessitating further research and development [53, 54].

8.4 Flow-Based Models

Flow-based models are a subset of generative models designed to learn exact likelihoods through invertible transformations between complex data distributions and simple base distributions (such as Gaussian distributions). The generative model architectures is illustrated in Fig. 7.

---

[1] There is a repository of GANs on https://github.com/hindupuravinash/the-gan-zoo

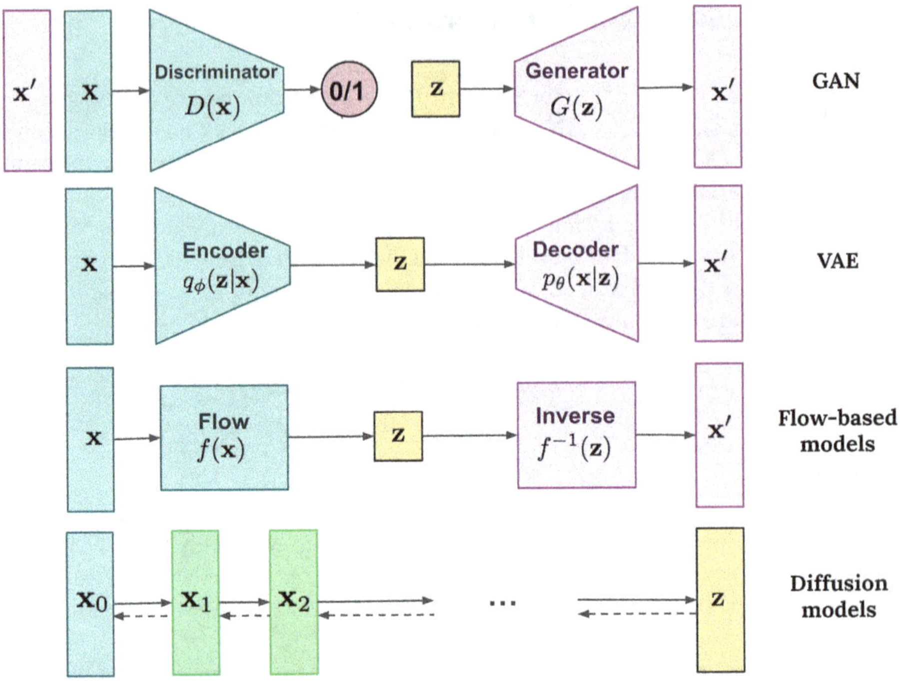

Fig. 7 Generative Models Architecture: GANs, VAEs, Flow-based models and Diffusion models

Applications
Flow-based models are utilized in medical imaging for tasks such as image reconstruction, feature disentanglement, and uncertainty quantification. They are particularly effective in inverse problems like low-dose CT and accelerated MRI, where they provide high-quality reconstructions by modeling complex data distributions [55]. Additionally, flow-based models like GLOWin are used to learn disentangled feature representations, which enhance interpretability and control over synthetic image generation [56].

Limitations Flow-based models can be computationally intensive due to their requirement for invertibility and complex architectures. This issue can limit scalability and application in real-time scenarios. Moreover, the choice of base distribution can significantly impact the quality of the generated images, necessitating careful selection and tuning [55].

8.5 Diffusion Models

Diffusion models represent a newer approach to generative modeling, particularly in medical imaging. Several diffusion-based generative models have been developed including diffusion probabilistic models [57], noise-conditioned score network [58], and Denoising Diffusion Probabilistic Models (DDPM) introduced by Ho et al. in 2020 [59]. These models work by defining a forward process that gradually adds noise to the data and a reverse process that learns to remove the noise to recover the original data distribution. The training of diffusion models involves learning the reverse process, which is typically parameterized by a neural network. Mathematically, given a data distribution $p(x)$, the forward process is defined as a sequence of noisy versions x_t for $t = 0,1,\ldots,T$ with $x_0 = x$. The reverse process is parameterized as a model $p_\theta(x_{t-1}|x_t)$ which attempts to denoise x_t to recover x_0. The objective function often involves minimizing the difference between the true reverse process and the model's output:

$$E_{x_0,t,\epsilon}\left[\left\|\epsilon - \epsilon_\theta\left(x_t,t\right)\right\|^2\right] \quad (11)$$

Where ϵ_θ is the neural network's estimate of the added noise at each step.

Applications
Diffusion models are used for high-quality image generation, segmentation, and anomaly detection in medical imaging. They are particularly effective in generating 3D medical images and enhancing image quality [60].

Limitations These models require significant computational resources and have limitations in controlling noise granularity, which can affect their generalizability across different anomaly types [61].

9 Recent Use Cases of GenAI in Medical Imaging

9.1 Image Generation and Synthesis

Recent improvements in GenAI applications for medical imaging primarily focus on enhancing diagnostic accuracy, addressing data scarcity, and facilitating training through image synthesis. Figure 8 presents some visual examples of generative models functionality in medical imaging. Popular frameworks include Deep Convolutional GAN (DCGAN), Laplacian GAN (LAPGAN), pix2pix, and CycleGAN, which have been enhanced with hybrid architectures for improved performance [31]. The Diffusion Deformable Model (DDM) is also a novel approach for generating 4D temporal medical images, such as cardiac MR images, by learning spatial deformation information [62]. The Light&Fast GAN model significantly improves the synthesis of high-fidelity liver tumor CT images, addressing issues such as imbalanced datasets in hepatocellular carcinoma (HCC) diagnosis. The model effectively simulates the morphological characteristics of liver tissues, achieving notable advances in image quality metrics and boosting classification accuracy by up to 34% [63]. The necessity of personalized synthetic data and standardized evaluation for clinical use is underscored in a recent comprehensive review

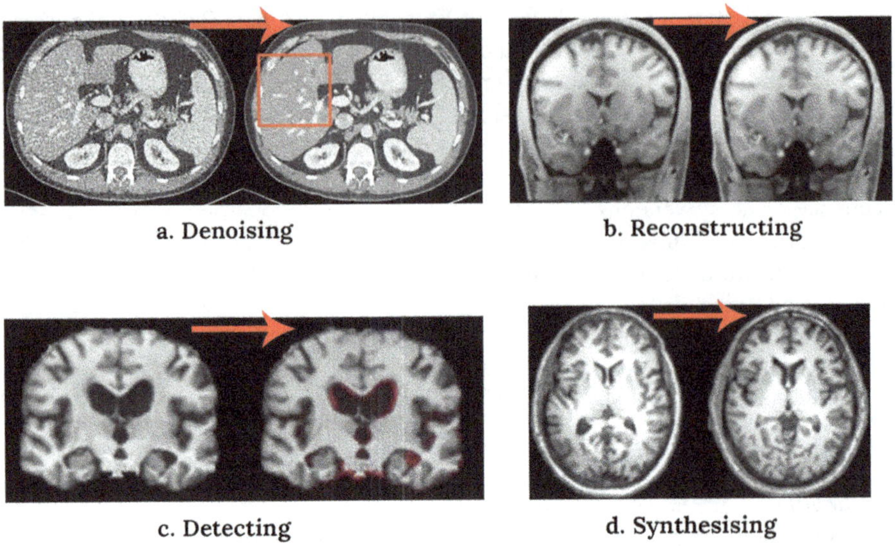

Fig. 8 Visual Examples of Generative Models Functionality in Medical Imaging. (**a**) Denoising [72], (**b**) Reconstructing [73], (**c**) Detecting [74], (**d**) Synthesising [75]

of generative models, which examines various kinds of medical modalities. The study highlights the potential of conditional models for enhanced synthetic data applications [64]. GANs are being leveraged to produce synthetic images for data augmentation, addressing the scarcity of medical image datasets, as exemplified by the Hierarchical GAN (HGAN), which enhances knee image synthesis for data enrichment [65].

Furthermore, the open-source GAN Image Synthesis Tool (GIST) provides scalable techniques for the generation of synthetic X-ray images, addressing privacy concerns and enhancing diagnostic algorithms in radiography [66]. Researchers also use GANs to generate controllable medical images, enabling attribute manipulation to meet specific research or clinical needs. This approach has been tested on modalities like mammograms, MRI, and CT [67].

9.2 Image Reconstruction and Enhancement

GANs are utilized to reconstruct medical images, including CT scans, by generating realistic images from randomized vectors. This approach seeks to produce high-quality images that closely resemble real data, enhancing diagnostic capabilities [68]. Super-Resolution Generative Adversarial Networks (SRGANs) are employed to enhance the resolution of medical images, which is crucial for telemedicine and diagnostics. SRGANs use a deep CNN generator and discriminator, guided by a perceptual loss function, to improve image clarity and detail [69]. Another approach is the Multi-Degradation-Adaptive Network, which enhances fundus images by dynamically addressing multiple degradation types. This technique significantly improves image quality by generating specific filters for each degradation mode, outperforming state-of-the-art methods in retinal image enhancement [70]. For domain adaptation in medical segmentation, the Dual Domain Distribution Disruption (DDSP) framework preserves anatomical structure while adapting across domains, resolving GAN instability issues. This framework excels in tasks like heart, brain, and prostate segmentation, achieving higher accuracy compared to previous methods [63]. Lastly, RetiGAN is a hybrid model combining Retinex theory and GANs that enhances medical images by improving contrast and texture details. This technique demonstrates potential in clinical diagnostics by significantly enhancing image quality metrics [71].

9.3 Image Segmentation and Anomaly Detection

A review of GAN applications in anomaly detection highlights their ability to generate new data, addressing the challenge of insufficient anomalous data. Common architectures include DCGANs and cGANs, with primary applications in medicine and surveillance [76]. For unsupervised anomaly detection, a fast residual attention network (F-UNetGAN) integrates U-Net-based discriminators to detect fine-grained anomalies, improving pixel-level accuracy and anomaly localization. The model excels at identifying anomalies in COVID-19 datasets and demonstrates its generalizability across several medical datasets [77]. Another approach, the Ano-cDiff model, employs a conditional-guided diffusion model to detect brain anomalies in multimodal MRI, offering a novel approach to pixel-level lesion prediction through adaptive prior correction. This model improves precision and dice scores for glioma segmentation tasks by a significant margin [78].

Furthermore, using ensembles of GANs can enhance stability and performance in anomaly detection tasks. By having multiple generators and discriminators interact GAN ensembles better model the distribution of normal data, leading to improved anomaly detection compared to single GAN models [79]. Lastly, Adjusted-LSTM GAN (ALGAN) is a model designed for time series anomaly detection, improving accuracy in both univariate and multivariate datasets. This approach demonstrates the versatility of GANs in different domains, including medical imaging [80].

10 Generative AI Platforms in Medical Imaging

Medical imaging plays a crucial role in healthcare. Health systems spend an estimated $65 billion each year on imaging [81], and approximately 80% of all hospital and health system visits include at least one imaging exam related to more than 23,000 conditions [82]. Regulatory permission has been granted to multiple generative AI applications in medical imaging, which are currently being utilized in clinical settings. These apps are essential for improving diagnostic accuracy, enhancing workflow efficiency, and supporting decision-making.

Nuance's PowerScribe with Precision Imaging Network (PIN)
This application incorporates AI-driven tools to automate radiological workflows. The PowerScribe platform, which seems to be utilized widely by more radiologists in the United States, has now integrated GenAI to assist with automatic report generation and structured data analysis. The Precision Imaging Network supports a unified point of access for AI models to automate tasks like organ segmentation, anomaly detection, and image classification across various modalities. This network is tightly integrated into hospital information systems, enabling radiologists to use real-time AI insights while maintaining compliance with regulatory standards.

Zebra Medical Vision's AI1
This solution offers several applications targeting specific medical conditions using generative models. Zebra's platform provides AI-based algorithms for the detection of diseases such as osteoporosis, emphysema, and fatty liver, analyzing data from imaging modalities like CT scans and X-rays. One of its key use cases is early detection of osteoporosis, where AI analyzes bone density scans and automatically generates risk assessments. The fatty liver diagnosis algorithm similarly uses CT images to evaluate liver conditions without requiring a biopsy.

Aidoc
Aidoc provides an AI-powered platform that analyzes medical images in real time to detect critical findings like brain hemorrhages, pulmonary embolisms, and strokes. The tool assists radiologists by flagging urgent cases in their workflow, reducing diagnostic delays, and improving patient outcomes. Aidoc's platform integrates directly with hospital PACS (Picture Archiving and Communication Systems), automating the detection and triage of patients requiring immediate intervention. One of its recognized use cases is in stroke care, where the system automatically detects ischemic strokes from CT angiograms and alerts the care team.

Lunit INSIGHT
Lunit's AI-powered imaging solution focuses on detecting lung abnormalities such as nodules and tuberculosis from chest X-rays. Lunit INSIGHT, deployed in clinical environments globally, offers real-time image analysis and assists radiologists in interpreting challenging cases. This AI system is designed to detect anomalies in chest radiographs, providing a risk score and localization heatmaps to aid clinicians in identifying early signs of lung cancer.

Arterys
Arterys utilize AI to interpret medical images in cardiology and oncology. Its CardioAI and LungAI platforms focus on automating tasks such as the quantification of cardiac volumes, detecting pulmonary nodules, and characterizing lung lesions from MRI and CT scans. One key use case is cardiac MRI analysis, where

AI automates the segmentation of the heart and measures ejection fractions, reducing the time taken to generate diagnostic reports and ensuring consistency.

Qure.ai
Qure.ai's qER platform is designed for rapid diagnosis of head injuries by analyzing CT scans to detect critical conditions like bleeds and fractures. It flags urgent findings such as midline shifts or skull fractures, streamlining the workflow in emergency departments. This AI application plays a critical role in trauma care by aiding clinicians in prioritizing patients who need urgent surgical intervention.

Viz.ai
Another significant application is Viz.ai, which focuses on stroke detection. Its AI algorithms analyze CT angiograms to detect large vessel occlusions (LVO) in stroke patients and alert specialists in real time. Viz.ai's LVO Stroke Platform integrates with hospital communication systems, helping ensure that stroke patients receive timely treatment, which is critical for improving survival rates and reducing long-term disability.

Subtle Medical
Subtle Medical provides AI software that enhances imaging workflows by reducing scan times and improving image quality in MRI and PET. SubtleMR and SubtlePET use AI to denoise and improve the resolution of low-dose scans. This results in faster scans with lower radiation exposure, making the technology valuable for pediatric imaging and routine diagnostic scans.

These tools demonstrate the practical applications of generative AI in medical imaging. They not only enhance diagnostic capabilities but also address challenges like data scarcity and improving access to AI models across clinical settings. The ongoing advancements in this space hold the potential to improve patient outcomes, reduce diagnostic errors, and optimize treatment planning. Table 2 summarizing some of the most popular regulatory-approved GenAI applications in medical imaging, including their specific use cases.

11 Python for Generative Models in Medical Imaging

Python tools have become increasingly important for implementing generative models. Here, we focus on key Python-based libraries and frameworks designed to utilize generative models specifically for medical imaging. These tools are essential for integrating GenAI into medical workflows, where the challenges of data scarcity, multimodality, and high dimensionality make traditional approaches less sufficient.

MONAI
Medical Open Network for AI (MONAI) [83] is a deep learning library built explicitly for medical imaging tasks and provides flexible tools for training models that can enhance, reconstruct, or generate medical images.

Table 2 Popular Generative AI Platforms in Medical Imaging

Platforms	Focus Area	Use Case	Key Features
Nuance PowerScribe	Radiology	Automating radiology report generation and real-time image analysis	Integration with hospital systems for workflow automation
Zebra Medical Vision (AI1)	Multi-modality imaging	Detects diseases like osteoporosis, cardiovascular conditions	AI algorithms for early disease detection and personalized risk assessments
Aidoc	Critical findings detection	Triage of brain hemorrhages, pulmonary embolisms, and strokes	Real-time flagging of urgent cases in radiology workflows
Lunit INSIGHT	Chest X-ray analysis	Detecting lung nodules, tuberculosis, and early-stage lung cancer	Real-time analysis with risk scoring and abnormality localization
Arterys	Cardiology, oncology	Cardiac MRI segmentation, lung nodule detection	Automated quantification of heart and lung metrics
Qure.ai (qER)	Head injury detection	Analyzes CT scans for bleeds, fractures, and midline shifts	Real-time trauma care prioritization in emergency departments
Viz.ai	Stroke detection	Detects large vessel occlusions in stroke patients from CT angiograms	Automated notifications to stroke specialists for timely intervention
Subtle Medical (SubtleMR, SubtlePET)	MRI, PET imaging enhancement	Reduces scan time and improves image resolution in MRI and PET	Denoising low-dose scans to reduce patient radiation exposure

- Advanced Transformations: MONAI excels in applying complex spatial and intensity-based transformations to medical images, which are essential when training GANs and VAEs to generate synthetic data. The library's augmentation capabilities are vital for creating diverse training datasets, especially when working with limited data.
- Pre-trained Models for Generative Tasks: MONAI includes pre-trained models for tasks like medical image segmentation and reconstruction. This is particularly useful for GenAI tasks such as cross-modality synthesis (e.g., MRI-to-CT generation) [84].
- Integration with PyTorch: MONAI is built on PyTorch and integrates easily with other generative models like StyleGAN, CycleGAN, or pix2pix. This makes it highly suitable for applications such as image translation between different medical imaging modalities or noise reduction in low-dose scans.

TorchIO

TorchIO [85] is built on PyTorch to work with 3D medical images, making it ideal for volumetric datasets such as MRI or CT scans. While it is primarily used for preprocessing and augmentation, it is highly complementary to GenAI workflows.

- Patch-Based Processing: In 3D data, training generative models like GANs or VAEs can be computationally intensive. TorchIO offers patch-based processing, making it feasible to generate synthetic medical images from smaller, localized regions while maintaining high anatomical detail.
- Advanced Data Augmentation: The library includes robust spatial transformations that are crucial for increasing dataset diversity when training generative models. These transformations help GANs and VAEs generalize better, allowing the generation of anatomically plausible synthetic images.

Medigan

Medigan is an open-source Python library specifically designed for generative models in medical imaging [86]. Its architecture is built to standardize the integration of generative models and facilitate reproducibility in synthetic image generation, especially in healthcare contexts. Medigan encapsulates several pre-trained generative models and provides an easy interface for training, evaluating, and fine-tuning them on medical datasets.

- Centralized Repository of GAN Models: Medigan provides a repository of pre-trained GAN architectures (DCGAN, CycleGAN, StyleGAN) tailored for specific medical imaging tasks like generating synthetic MRI or CT scans and performing cross-modality image translation. This reduces the time needed to deploy models and allows for easy adaptation to various clinical needs.
- Customization and Adaptability: Medigan supports model customization, allowing users to tweak GAN architectures and training pipelines. For example, users can adapt existing GANs for tasks like lesion detection, anomaly detection, or noise removal from medical images.
- Clinical Utility: Medigan's focus on healthcare ensures compatibility with DICOM data and support for privacy-preserving machine learning. Researchers can also use the platform to generate synthetic data for rare diseases, which can augment clinical training datasets and improve model robustness.

Pythae

Pythae is a Python library designed to work with autoencoders, particularly variational autoencoders (VAEs) and their variants [87]. Although Pythae is not exclusively built for medical imaging, its flexible and modular design makes it highly relevant in this domain, where VAEs are utilized for tasks such as image reconstruction, anomaly detection, and data compression.

- Wide Range of Models: Pythae supports a variety of VAE architectures, including β-VAE, conditional VAE (CVAE), and others, which are helpful in generating images conditioned on specific variables like pathology or organ type.
- Latent Space Manipulation: One of the strengths of Pythae is the ability to explore and manipulate latent spaces. This feature is critical in applications such as disease progression modeling or anomaly detection, where understanding variations within the latent space of medical data can lead to important clinical insights.

- Flexible Training and Modular Design: Pythae's modular design allows for extensive customization, making it easier to apply VAE-based models to specific medical imaging tasks. Researchers can modify the latent space dimensions or incorporate custom loss functions to tailor the models to specialized medical imaging problems.

NVIDIA Clara

NVIDIA Clara is a versatile AI toolkit developed for healthcare and medical imaging applications. It integrates advanced AI capabilities with GPU acceleration, offering a suite of tools optimized for training and deploying deep learning models, including generative models. Its compatibility with medical standards like DICOM makes it an essential platform for both research and clinical applications.

- Cross-Modality Synthesis and Image Quality Enhancement: GANs like CycleGAN enable translation between imaging modalities (e.g., MRI to CT), which is crucial when certain modalities are unavailable. Additionally, these models improve image quality by removing noise, filling in gaps, or increasing resolution, which enhances diagnostic accuracy, especially for low-quality scans like low-dose CTs or noisy MRIs.
- Privacy-Preserving Synthetic Data: Clara generates synthetic medical data that mirrors real patient data, enabling training and sharing of AI models without compromising patient privacy.
- Anomaly Detection: Clara's GANs help identify anomalies by learning patterns in medical images and detecting deviations, assisting in the early detection of conditions like tumors or lesions that might be missed through traditional imaging methods.
- Transfer Learning for Accelerated Model Development: Clara supports transfer learning, allowing researchers to fine-tune pre-trained generative models for specific datasets. This reduces the need for extensively annotated datasets and accelerates the development and deployment of specialized models in clinical settings.

12 Medical Multimodal LLMs

While Large Language Models (LLMs) are primarily designed for text-based tasks, their utility in medical imaging arises from their ability to interpret and generate descriptive language regarding visual data. LLMs can process large datasets of radiological reports, synthesize findings, and generate human-like diagnostic recommendations. Vision-Language Models (VLMs) integrate visual and textual data, allowing for more comprehensive analysis and interpretation of medical images. These models can synthesize realistic medical images and assist in tasks such as image classification and segmentation.

Recent advancements in foundation models have drawn attention to medical AI system development [88]. These models are designed to generalize across diverse tasks and domains, which positions them as a powerful tool for solving complex medical problems. Multimodal Large Language Models (MLLMs) integrate multiple forms of data, ranging from medical images to electronic health records (EHRs) and clinical findings, to offer comprehensive diagnostic, therapeutic, and patient management solutions. Developments in large models have produced advanced MLLMs, such as Med-Gemini, which showcases robust multimodal processing abilities [89]. Med-Gemini and similar models are designed to handle various types of medical information simultaneously, allowing clinicians to interact with the data more intuitively and efficiently. For instance, an MLLM could analyze an MRI scan, consider a patient's lab results, and incorporate a physician's notes to provide a comprehensive diagnostic report. This multimodal synthesis not only enhances diagnostic precision but also makes the results more interpretable for clinicians, thereby fostering trust in AI-driven medical decision-making [90].

13 Conclusion

In conclusion, the integration of Generative AI in medical imaging marks a transformative leap in both technology and healthcare. As we have explored, AI-driven advancements, particularly generative models such as GANs, VAEs, and diffusion models, hold significant potential in revolutionizing image synthesis, data augmentation, and anomaly detection. These approaches provide innovative solutions for longstanding challenges in the field, including the scarcity of annotated medical data, limitations in diagnostic accuracy, and the need for improved image quality in modalities such as MRI, CT, and PET.

Generative models have demonstrated their utility across various applications, such as cross-modality image synthesis, super-resolution, and denoising, which not only enhance image analysis but also optimize clinical workflows by enabling faster, more accurate diagnostics. The clinical application of these technologies, as illustrated by regulatory-approved AI tools shows their increasing relevance in real-world healthcare environments, particularly in critical settings like stroke detection and lung cancer screening.

Despite these advancements, challenges remain, including issues related to data privacy, algorithmic bias, and the resource-intensive nature of AI model training. Moreover, the implementation of AI systems in clinical settings necessitates significant infrastructure, regulatory approvals, and collaboration between interdisciplinary teams of clinicians, AI researchers, and engineers. As AI continues to evolve, addressing these challenges will be crucial to maximizing its impact on medical imaging and ensuring its ethical, reliable, and effective use.

14 Future Research

A critical area for future research in GenAI within medical imaging is improving the generalization of models across different medical centers, populations, and imaging modalities. Many AI models, while highly accurate in controlled environments, struggle with performance when exposed to real-world variability in patient demographics, imaging equipment, or clinical practices. Addressing this requires creating more robust algorithms capable of adapting to diverse clinical settings. Another important research focus is minimizing computational costs. Training large-scale generative models, especially those that leverage deep learning architectures, demands immense computational resources.

Future research should prioritize the integration of GenAI with other emerging technologies to create holistic healthcare systems. Combining medical imaging data with other health records, and clinical notes through advanced AI systems could open new frontiers in personalized medicine, early disease detection, and treatment planning. This multimodal approach will likely be pivotal in advancing AI-driven diagnostics and care pathways.

References

1. Goodfellow I, Pouget-Abadie J, Mirza M, Xu B, Warde-Farley D, Ozair S, et al. Generative adversarial nets. In: Advances in neural information processing systems, vol. 27; 2014.
2. Mirza M, Osindero S. Conditional generative adversarial nets. ArXiv.org; 2014. https://arxiv.org/abs/1411.1784.
3. Zhu JY, Park T, Isola P, Efros AA. Unpaired image-to-image translation using cycle-consistent adversarial networks. In: Proceedings of the IEEE international conference on computer vision; 2017. p. 2223–32.
4. Zhang H, Xu T, Li H, Zhang S, Wang X, Huang X, Metaxas DN. Stackgan: text to photo-realistic image synthesis with stacked generative adversarial networks. In: Proceedings of the IEEE international conference on computer vision; 2017. p. 5907–15.
5. Karras T, Aila T, Laine S, Lehtinen J. Progressive growing of GANs for improved quality, stability, and variation. ArXiv.org; 2017. https://arxiv.org/abs/1710.10196v3.
6. Karras T, Laine S, Aila T. A style-based generator architecture for generative adversarial networks. In: Proceedings of the IEEE/CVF conference on computer vision and pattern recognition; 2019. p. 4401–10.
7. Tay YX, Kothan S, Kada S, Cai S, Lai CWK. Challenges and optimization strategies in medical imaging service delivery during COVID-19. World J Radiol. 2021;13(5):102–21. https://doi.org/10.4329/wjr.v13.i5.102.
8. Khalifa M, Albadawy M. AI in diagnostic imaging: revolutionising accuracy and efficiency. Comput Methods Programs Biomed Update. 2024;5:100146. https://doi.org/10.1016/j.cmpbup.2024.100146.
9. Mahant PD. A Radiologist's art in CT images. Int J User-Driven Healthcare. 2013;3(4):61–6. https://doi.org/10.4018/ijudh.2013100109.
10. Frush D, Denham CR, Goske MJ, Brink JA, Morin RL, Mills TT, Butler PF, McCollough C, Miller DL. Radiation protection and dose monitoring in medical imaging: a journey from awareness, through accountability, ability and action…but where will we arrive? J Patient Saf. 2013;9(4):232–8. https://doi.org/10.1097/PTS.0b013e3182a8c2c4.
11. Faragallah OS, El-Hoseny H, El-Shafai W, El-Rahman WA, El-Sayed HS, El-Rabaie E-SM, El-Samie FEA, Geweid GGN. A comprehensive survey analysis for present solutions of medical image fusion and future directions. IEEE Access. 2021;9:11358–71. https://doi.org/10.1109/access.2020.3048315.
12. Tourassi GD. Computer assisted radiology (CAR). In: Wiley Encyclopedia of biomedical engineering; 2006. https://doi.org/10.1002/9780471740360.ebs1432.

13. Nsoesie EO. Evaluating artificial intelligence applications in clinical settings. JAMA Netw Open. 2018;1(5):e182658. https://doi.org/10.1001/jamanetworkopen.2018.2658.
14. Joshi G, Jain A, Araveeti SR, Adhikari S, Garg H, Bhandari M. FDA-approved artificial intelligence and machine learning (AI/ML)-enabled medical devices: an updated landscape. Electronics. 2024;13(3):498. https://doi.org/10.3390/electronics13030498.
15. Bushberg JT, Boone JM. The essential physics of medical imaging. Lippincott Williams & Wilkins; 2011.
16. Bhagat AP, Atique M. Medical images: Formats, compression techniques and DICOM image retrieval a survey. International conference on devices, circuits and systems, 2012. https://doi.org/10.1109/icdcsyst.2012.6188698.
17. Polzehl J, Tabelow K. Medical imaging data formats. Use R! 2019:15–24. https://doi.org/10.1007/978-3-030-29184-6_3.
18. Larobina M, Murino L. Medical image file formats. J Digit Imaging. 2014;27(2):200–6. https://doi.org/10.1007/s10278-013-9657-9.
19. Parikh SS, Ruiz D, Kalva H, Fernandez-Escribano G, Adzic V. High bit-depth medical image compression with HEVC. IEEE J Biomed Health Inform. 2018;22(2):552–60. https://doi.org/10.1109/jbhi.2017.2660482.
20. Buchanan BG, Shortliffe EH. Rule based expert systems: the mycin experiments of the stanford heuristic programming project (the Addison-Wesley series in artificial intelligence). Addison-Wesley Longman Publishing Co., Inc.; 1984.
21. Pires PB, Santos JD, Pereira IV. Artificial neural networks: history and state of the art. In: Khosrow-Pour M, D.B.A, editors. Encyclopedia of information science and technology. 6th ed. Advance online publication; 2025. https://doi.org/10.4018/978-1-6684-7366-5.ch037.
22. Cheng PM, Montagnon E, Yamashita R, Pan I, Cadrin-Chênevert A, Perdigón Romero F, Chartrand G, Kadoury S, Tang A. Deep learning: an update for radiologists. Radiographics. 2021;41(5):1427–45. https://doi.org/10.1148/rg.2021200210.
23. Shurrab S, Duwairi R. Self-supervised learning methods and applications in medical imaging analysis: a survey. PeerJ Comput Sci. 2022;8:e1045. https://doi.org/10.7717/peerj-cs.1045.
24. Taher MRH, Haghighi F, Gotway MB, Liang J. Caid: context-aware instance discrimination for self-supervised learning in medical imaging. In: International conference on medical imaging with deep learning. PMLR; 2022, December. p. 535–51.
25. Zhang J, Xie Y, Wu Q, Xia Y. Medical image classification using synergic deep learning. Med Image Anal. 2019;54:10–9. https://doi.org/10.1016/j.media.2019.02.010.
26. Shou Y, Meng T, Ai W, Xie C, Liu H, Wang Y. Object detection in medical images based on hierarchical transformer and mask mechanism; 2022. p. 1–12. https://doi.org/10.1155/2022/5863782.
27. Liu Y, Li Y, Jiang M, Wang S, Ye S, Walsh S, Yang G. SOCR-YOLO: small objects detection algorithm in medical images. Int J Imaging Syst Technol. 2024;34(4) https://doi.org/10.1002/ima.23130.
28. Guo Z, Li X, Huang H, Guo N, Li Q. Deep learning-based image segmentation on multimodal medical imaging. IEEE Trans Radiat Plasma Med Sci. 2019;3(2):162–9. https://doi.org/10.1109/TRPMS.2018.2890359.
29. Zhang L, Deng X, Lu Y. Segment Anything Model (SAM) for medical image segmentation: a preliminary review. In: 2023 IEEE international conference on bioinformatics and biomedicine (BIBM). IEEE; 2023, December. p. 4187–94. https://doi.org/10.1109/bibm58861.2023.10386032.
30. Mohammed HA, Hassan MA. The image registration techniques for medical imaging (MRI-CT). American Journal of Biomedical Engineering. 2016;6(2):53–8.
31. Singh NK, Raza K. Medical image generation using generative adversarial networks: a review. In: Health informatics: a computational perspective in healthcare; 2021. p. 77–96. https://doi.org/10.1007/978-981-15-9735-0_5.
32. Kidder BL. Advanced image generation for cancer using diffusion models. BioRxiv (Cold Spring Harbor Laboratory); 2023. https://doi.org/10.1101/2023.08.18.553859.

33. Adams LC, Busch F, Truhn D, Makowski MR, Aerts HJWL, Bressem KK. What does DALL-E 2 know about radiology? J Med Internet Res. 2023;25:e43110. https://doi.org/10.2196/43110.
34. Santoro A, Raposo D, Barrett DG, Malinowski M, Pascanu R, Battaglia P, Lillicrap T. A simple neural network module for relational reasoning. Advances in neural information processing systems. 2017;30. https://arxiv.org/abs/1706.01427.
35. Van Den Oord A, Kalchbrenner N, Kavukcuoglu K. Pixel recurrent neural networks. In: International conference on machine learning. PMLR; 2016, June. p. 1747–56.
36. Van den Oord A, Kalchbrenner N, Espeholt L, Vinyals O, Graves A, Kavukcuoglu K. Conditional image generation with pixelcnn decoders. Advances in neural information processing systems. 2016;29. https://arxiv.org/abs/1606.05328v2.
37. Kingma DP, Welling M. Auto-encoding variational bayes. ArXiv.org; 2013. https://arxiv.org/abs/1312.6114.
38. Wei R, Mahmood A. Recent advances in variational autoencoders with representation learning for biomedical informatics: a survey. IEEE Access. 2021;9:4939–56. https://doi.org/10.1109/access.2020.3048309.
39. Akrami H, Joshi AA, Aydore S, Leahy RM. Addressing variance shrinkage in variational autoencoders using quantile regression. ArXiv.org; 2020. https://arxiv.org/abs/2010.09042.
40. Zhou L, Deng W, Wu X. Unsupervised anomaly localization using VAE and beta-VAE. ArXiv.org; 2020. https://arxiv.org/abs/2005.10686v1.
41. Musalamadugu TS, Kannan H. Generative AI for medical imaging analysis and applications. Future Medicine AI. 2023;1(2). https://doi.org/10.2217/fmai-2023-0004.
42. Illimoottil M, Ginat D. Recent advances in deep learning and medical imaging for head and neck cancer treatment: MRI, CT, and PET scans. Cancers. 2023;15(13):3267. https://doi.org/10.3390/cancers15133267.
43. Rahman MM, Shokouhmand S, Bhatt S, Faezipour M. Mist: medical image segmentation transformer with convolutional attention mixing (cam) decoder. In: Proceedings of the IEEE/CVF winter conference on applications of computer vision; 2024. p. 404–13.
44. Koohi-Moghadam M, Bae KT. Generative AI in medical imaging: applications, challenges, and ethics. Journal of Medical Systems. 2023;47(1):94. https://doi.org/10.1007/s10916-023-01987-4.
45. Wang Y, Zhou C, Ying L, Chan HP, Lee E, Chughtai A, Hadjiiski LM, Kazerooni EA. Enhancing early lung cancer diagnosis: predicting lung nodule progression in follow-up low-dose CT scan with deep generative model. Cancers. 2024;16(12):2229. https://doi.org/10.3390/cancers16122229.
46. Salama WM, Shokry A, Aly MH. A generalized framework for lung cancer classification based on deep generative models. Multimed Tools Appl. 2022;81(23):32705–22. https://doi.org/10.1007/s11042-022-13005-9.
47. Tan J, Jing L, Huo Y, Li L, Akin O, Tian Y. LGAN: Lung segmentation in CT scans using generative adversarial network. Computerized Medical Imaging and Graphics. 2021;87:101817. https://doi.org/10.1016/j.compmedimag.2020.101817.
48. Xu Z, Qi C, Xu G. Semi-supervised attention-guided cyclegan for data augmentation on medical images. In: 2019 IEEE international conference on bioinformatics and biomedicine (BIBM). IEEE; 2019, November. p. 563–8. https://doi.org/10.1109/bibm47256.2019.8982932.
49. Qi C, Chen J, Xu G, Xu Z, Lukasiewicz T, Liu Y. SAG-GAN: semi-supervised attention-guided GANs for data augmentation on medical images. ArXiv:2011.07534 [Cs, Eess]; 2020. https://arxiv.org/abs/2011.07534.
50. Lin S, Qin F, Li Y, Bly RA, Moe KS, Hannaford B. Lc-gan: image-to-image translation based on generative adversarial network for endoscopic images. In: 2020 IEEE/RSJ international conference on intelligent robots and systems (IROS). IEEE; 2020, October. p. 2914–20. https://doi.org/10.1109/iros45743.2020.9341556.
51. Desalegn L, Jifara W. HARA-GAN: hybrid attention and relative average discriminator based generative adversarial network for MR image reconstruction. IEEE Access. 2024; https://doi.org/10.1109/access.2024.3364699.

52. Huang Z, Zhang J, Zhang Y, Shan H. DU-GAN: generative adversarial networks with dual-domain U-net-based discriminators for low-dose CT denoising. IEEE Trans Instrum Meas. 2022;71:1–12. https://doi.org/10.1109/tim.2021.3128703.
53. Gong M, Chen S, Chen Q, Zeng Y, Zhang Y. Generative adversarial networks in medical image processing. Curr Pharm Des. 2020;26 https://doi.org/10.2174/1381612826666201125110710.
54. Liu J, Li K, Dong H, Han Y, Li R. Medical image processing based on generative adversarial networks: a systematic review. Curr Med Imag Rev. 2023;20 https://doi.org/10.2174/0115734056258198230920042358.
55. Denker A, Schmidt M, Leuschner J, Maass P. Conditional invertible neural networks for medical imaging. J Imag. 2021;7(11):243. https://doi.org/10.3390/jimaging7110243.
56. Sankar A, Keicher M, Eisawy R, Parida A, Pfister F, Kim ST, Navab N. GLOWin: a flow-based invertible generative framework for learning disentangled feature representations in medical images. ArXiv.org; 2021. https://arxiv.org/abs/2103.10868v1.
57. Sohl-Dickstein J, Weiss E, Maheswaranathan N, Ganguli S. Deep unsupervised learning using nonequilibrium thermodynamics. In: International conference on machine learning. PMLR; 2015, June. p. 2256–65.
58. Song Y, Ermon S. Generative modeling by estimating gradients of the data distribution. Advances in neural information processing systems. 2019;32.
59. Ho J, Jain A, Abbeel P. Denoising diffusion probabilistic models. Advances in neural information processing systems. 2020;33:6840–51.
60. Bieder F, Wolleb J, Durrer A, Sandkühler R, Cattin PC. Diffusion models for memory-efficient processing of 3D medical images. ArXiv.org; 2023. https://arxiv.org/abs/2303.15288.
61. Bercea CI, Neumayr M, Rueckert D, Schnabel JA. Mask, stitch, and re-sample: enhancing robustness and generalizability in anomaly detection through automatic diffusion models. ArXiv.org; 2023. https://arxiv.org/abs/2305.19643.
62. Kim B, Ye JC. Diffusion deformable model for 4D temporal medical image generation. In: International conference on medical image computing and computer-assisted intervention. Cham: Springer Nature Switzerland; 2022, September. p. 539–48. https://doi.org/10.1007/978-3-031-16431-6_51.
63. Zheng Z, Wang M, Fan C, Wang C, He X, He X. Light&Fast generative adversarial network for high-fidelity CT image synthesis of liver tumor. Comput Methods Prog Biomed. 2024;108252 https://doi.org/10.1016/j.cmpb.2024.108252.
64. Ibrahim M, Khalil YA, Amirrajab S, Sun C, Breeuwer M, Pluim J, Elen B, Ertaylan G, Dumontier M. Generative AI for synthetic data across multiple medical modalities: a systematic review of recent developments and challenges. ArXiv.org; 2024. https://arxiv.org/abs/2407.00116v2
65. Wen Y, Mei Z, Qi C. Generative Adversarial Networks (GANs) for image synthesis and augmentation. In: 2024 IEEE 4th international conference on electronic technology, communication and information (ICETCI). IEEE; 2024, May. p. 1244–9. https://doi.org/10.1109/ICETCI61221.2024.10594365.
66. McNulty JR, Kho L, Case AL, Slater D, Abzug JM, Russell SA. Synthetic medical imaging generation with generative adversarial networks for plain radiographs. Appl Sci. 2024;14(15):6831. https://doi.org/10.3390/app14156831.
67. Ren Z, Stella XY, Whitney D. Controllable medical image generation via GAN. J Percept Imag. 2022;5:0005021. https://doi.org/10.2352/j.percept.imaging.2022.5.000502.
68. Dang N, Khurana M, Tiwari S. MirGAN: medical image reconstruction using generative adversarial networks. In: 2020 5th international conference on computing, communication and security (ICCCS). IEEE; 2020, October. p. 1–5. https://doi.org/10.1109/ICCCS49678.2020.9277127.
69. Varshitha S, Lavanya N, Shirisha M, Manmatti S, Kp AR, Gowrishankar S. Enhancing medical imaging resolution: exploring SRGAN for high-quality medical image reconstruction. In: 2024 IEEE international conference for women in innovation, technology &

entrepreneurship (ICWITE). IEEE; 2024, February. p. 1–8. https://doi.org/10.1109/ICWITE59797.2024.10503215.
70. Guo R, Xu Y, Tompkins A, Pagnucco M, Song Y. Multi-degradation-adaptation network for fundus image enhancement with degradation representation learning. Med Image Anal. 2024;97:103273. https://doi.org/10.1016/j.media.2024.103273.
71. Huang Z, Wang S, Hu H, Xu Y. RetiGAN: a hybrid image enhancement method for medical images. In: 2024 5th international conference on computer vision, image and deep learning (CVIDL). IEEE; 2024, April. p. 25–9. https://doi.org/10.1109/CVIDL62147.2024.10603883.
72. Shan H, Zhang Y, Yang Q, Kruger U, Kalra MK, Sun L, et al. 3-D convolutional encoder-decoder network for low-dose CT via transfer learning from a 2-D trained network. IEEE Trans Med Imaging. 2018;37(6):1522–34. https://doi.org/10.1109/TMI.2018.2832217.
73. Chen Y, Shi F, Christodoulou AG, Xie Y, Zhou Z, Li D. Efficient and accurate MRI super-resolution using a generative adversarial network and 3D multi-level densely connected network. In: International conference on medical image computing and computer-assisted intervention. Cham: Springer International Publishing; 2018, September. p. 91–9. https://doi.org/10.1007/978-3-030-00928-1_11.
74. Baumgartner CF, Koch LM, Tezcan KC, Ang JX, Konukoglu E. Visual feature attribution using wasserstein gans. In: Proceedings of the IEEE conference on computer vision and pattern recognition; 2018. p. 8309–19.
75. Bermudez C, Plassard AJ, Davis LT, Newton AT, Resnick SM, Landman BA. Learning implicit brain MRI manifolds with deep learning. In: Medical imaging 2018: image processing, vol. 10574. SPIE; 2018, March. p. 408–14. https://doi.org/10.1117/12.2293515.
76. Sabuhi M, Zhou M, Bezemer CP, Musilek P. Applications of generative adversarial networks in anomaly detection: a systematic literature review. IEEE Access. 2021;9:161003–29. https://doi.org/10.1109/ACCESS.2021.3131949.
77. Nafti N, Besbes O, Abdallah AB, Vacavant A, Bedoui MH. A fast residual attention network for fine-grained unsupervised anomaly detection and localization. Appl Soft Comput. 2024;165:112066. https://doi.org/10.1016/j.asoc.2024.112066.
78. Chen X, Peng Y. Counterfactual condition diffusion with continuous prior adaptive correction for anomaly detection in multimodal brain MRI. Expert Syst Appl. 2024;124295 https://doi.org/10.1016/j.eswa.2024.124295.
79. Han X, Chen X, Liu LP. Gan ensemble for anomaly detection. In: Proceedings of the AAAI conference on artificial intelligence, vol. 35, No. 5; 2021, May. p. 4090–7. https://doi.org/10.1609/aaai.v35i5.16530.
80. Bashar MA, Nayak R. ALGAN: time series anomaly detection with adjusted-LSTM GAN. ArXiv.org; 2023. https://arxiv.org/abs/2308.06663v2.
81. Smith-Bindman R, Miglioretti DL, Johnson E, Lee C, Feigelson HS, Flynn M, et al. Use of diagnostic imaging studies and associated radiation exposure for patients enrolled in large integrated health care systems, 1996-2010. JAMA. 2012;307(22):2400–9. https://doi.org/10.1001/jama.2012.5960.
82. Healthcare D. Healthcare Analytics & Provider Data | Definitive Healthcare, n.d. https://www.definitivehc.com/
83. Jorge CM, Li W, Brown R, Ma N, Kerfoot E, Wang Y, Murrey B, Myronenko A, Zhao C, Yang D, Nath V, He Y, Xu Z, Hatamizadeh A, Myronenko A, Zhu W, Liu Y, Zheng M, Tang Y, Yang I. MONAI: an open-source framework for deep learning in healthcare. ArXiv.org; 2022. https://arxiv.org/abs/2211.02701v1.
84. Walter, Graham MS, Kerfoot E, Tudosiu P-D, Dafflon J, Fernandez V, Sanchez P, Wolleb J, Pedro, Patel A, Chung H, Zhao C, Peng W, Liu Z, Mei X, Lucena O, Ye JC, Tsaftaris SA, Dogra P, Feng A. Generative AI for medical imaging: extending the MONAI framework. ArXiv.org; 2023. https://arxiv.org/abs/2307.15208v1.
85. Pérez-García F, Sparks R, Ourselin S. TorchIO: a Python library for efficient loading, preprocessing, augmentation and patch-based sampling of medical images in deep learning. Comput Methods Prog Biomed. 2021;208:106236. https://doi.org/10.1016/j.cmpb.2021.106236.

86. Osuala R, Skorupko G, Lazrak N, Garrucho L, García E, Joshi S, et al. medigan: a Python library of pretrained generative models for medical image synthesis. J Med Imag. 2023;10(6):061403. https://doi.org/10.1117/1.jmi.10.6.061403.
87. Chadebec C, Vincent L, Allassonnière S. Pythae: Unifying generative autoencoders in python-a benchmarking use case. Advances in Neural Information Processing Systems. 2022;35:21575–89.
88. Zhang S, Xu Y, Usuyama N, Xu H, Bagga J, Tinn R, Preston S, Rao R, Wei M, Valluri N, Wong C, Tupini A, Wang Y, Mazzola M, Shukla S, Liden L, Gao J, Lungren MP, Naumann T, Wang S. BiomedCLIP: a multimodal biomedical foundation model pretrained from fifteen million scientific image-text pairs. ArXiv.org; 2024. https://arxiv.org/abs/2303.00915v2.
89. Saab K, Tu T, Weng W-H, Tanno R, Stutz D, Wulczyn E, Zhang F, Strother T, Park C, Vedadi E, Chaves JZ, Hu S-Y, Schaekermann M, Kamath A, Cheng Y, David B, Cheung C, Mustafa B, Palepu A, McDuff D. Capabilities of Gemini models in medicine. ArXiv.org; 2024. https://arxiv.org/abs/2404.18416v2.
90. Zhang Y, Pan Y, Zhong T, Dong P, Xie K, Liu Y, et al. Potential of multimodal large language models for data mining of medical images and free-text reports. Meta-Radiol. 2024;100103 https://doi.org/10.1016/j.metrad.2024.100103.

Generative AI in Pandemic Prediction

Parisa Tavana and Mohammad ZareiNejad

1 Introduction

A global and widespread pandemic is defined as "the outbreak of a new disease worldwide." When a new disease first appears, most of us lack the natural immunity to combat it. This can lead to sudden and sometimes rapid spread of the disease among people in communities and around the world. On the other hand, generative artificial intelligence can be used to create more realistic and consequently more reliable models of how a pandemic spread. This approach can simultaneously consider human behavior, environmental factors, and virus characteristics to provide crucial information. This chapter addresses the impact of generative AI on pandemic prediction and management, introduces new approaches, and discusses the challenges and limitations in this field.

Major pandemics such as the plague and COVID-19 have previously affected the economy and human health. A study [1] states that many infectious diseases leading to pandemics are caused by zoonotic pathogens, which have been transmitted to humans due to increased contact with animals through farming, hunting, and global trade activities. Understanding the mechanisms of pathogen transmission to humans has also enabled the development of infection prevention and control methods. Over the centuries, the implementation of public health measures such as isolation, quarantine, and border control has helped contain the spread of contagious diseases and

P. Tavana (✉)
Department of Computer Engineering, Science and Research Branch, Islamic Azad University, Tehran, Iran
e-mail: parisa.tavana@srbiau.ac.ir

M. ZareiNejad
Department of Computer Engineering, South Tehran Branch, Islamic Azad University, Tehran, Iran
e-mail: St_m_zareinejad@azad.ac.ir

A. Zamanifar, M. Faezipour (eds.), *Application of Generative AI in Healthcare Systems*, https://doi.org/10.1007/978-3-031-82963-5_2

maintain societal structure. Pandemics disrupt our sense of reality and order, leading to changes in the way we store and process memories and experiences [2]. Additionally, pandemics have significantly shifted towards online education and learning [3]. Study [4] defines the interspecies transmission process of pathogens in five stages.

1. The pathogen exclusively infects animals under natural conditions.
2. The pathogen evolves to be transmissible to humans, but without sustained human-to-human transmission.
3. The pathogen experiences only a few cycles of secondary human-to-human transmission.
4. The disease exists in animals, but long sequences of secondary human-to-human transmission occur without involving an animal host.
5. The disease exclusively occurs in humans.

The terms endemic, outbreak, epidemic, and pandemic refer to the occurrence of a health condition compared to its expected rate and its spread across geographical areas [5]. An epidemic is an outbreak that spreads to larger geographical areas, while a pandemic is a global spread of an epidemic [1]. The use of these terms by official health agencies, scientists, and the media often seems contradictory [6]. For example, some argue that a high level of explosive spread is enough to declare a pandemic, while others believe that the severity of the infection should also be considered [7]. Study [8] states that defining the existence of a pandemic depends on the time, place, and size of the affected population. For instance, influenza is not considered a pandemic unless its spread is observed internationally in a highly concurrent pattern rather than being limited to expected seasonal outbreaks in different regions. It should be noted that since the next pandemic is most likely to be caused by influenza, this disease remains a top public health threat in the region. The WHE continues to collaborate with member states to strengthen their capacities for prevention, surveillance, and response to both seasonal and zoonotic influenza with pandemic potential [9]. It should be noted that the spread of a pandemic, unlike most disasters, has predictable epidemiological models that provide a limited yet valuable time for forecasting, planning, and preparing as the pandemic approaches and progresses [2].

Despite the limited attention to the field of pandemics in research, this phenomenon has a profound impact on societies, mental health, and the economy. Following the COVID-19 pandemic, all countries are developing plans to gradually resume their economic and social activities, as the socio-economic situation has grown unstable [10]. Therefore, measuring the spread of disease during a pandemic is crucial for the precise and rapid implementation of various quarantine strategies to prevent the collapse of the medical system [11]. In theory, if everyone's movement is restricted and completely isolated, there is no chance of the virus being transmitted from one person to another. However, this would mean a significant economic loss as productivity and activities come to a halt [11]. Long-term isolation and separation from family and society can have profound effects on individuals even if they are merely isolated and not directly affected by the disease [2]. Ultimately, the discovery of microbial causes of diseases led to the production of vaccines and antisera against them and widespread diagnostic tests to study and monitor diseases at their sources [6].

In this chapter, we first review major pandemics such as the plague and COVID-19 and their impacts on societies and health. Then, we provide a brief introduction to generative artificial intelligence and its impact on the field of pandemics. Next, we introduce approaches to pandemic prediction and compare traditional models with AI-based generative models. Finally, by introducing the advantages and disadvantages of these approaches, we outline the future directions of this field. There are numerous examples of pandemic diseases in history, the most recent being the COVID-19 pandemic. To understand the problems and damages of pandemics, a summary of major pandemics up to the present time is provided below.

1.1 Justinian Plague

The plague in the Middle Ages caused brutal outbreaks, including the Justinian Plague and the "Black Death" [12]. Mortality estimates suggest that the Justinianic Plague (circa 541 to 750 AD) led to the deaths of tens of millions across the Mediterranean and Europe, contributing to the end of antiquity and the beginning of the Middle Ages [13]. The Justinian Plague originated in Egypt and spread throughout the Eastern Roman Empire and its neighbors [14]. The exact origin is unknown, but it likely reached Egypt via the Red Sea trade routes [15]. Like many pandemics, the Justinian Plague generally followed trade routes, facilitating the "exchange of contaminations as well as goods," and was thus particularly brutal for coastal cities [2]. During this pandemic, staple foods became scarce, and people died from starvation as well as the disease itself [16]. The impacts were extensive, affecting demography, the economy, craft production, agriculture, construction work, and foreign policy, devastating major cities and coastal trade centers, including the capital, where perhaps half the population perished [17]. After this event, the plague remained a recurring feature of the old world for centuries, deeply shaping its society, economy, and culture, with the Black Death marking the beginning of the "plague era" [15].

1.2 Black Death

The Black Death was the greatest population shock in European history [18]. Following the horrific outbreak in the 540 s, the plague remained endemic in Europe, the Mediterranean, and the Middle East for two centuries, regularly reappearing and causing terrible, though more localized, epidemics [15]. The mortality rate of the Black Death varied between regions, sometimes sparing sparsely populated rural areas but then decimating densely populated urban areas, where more than 50%, sometimes 60%, of the population perished [19]. Disruptions in trade networks and increased transaction costs hit the most commercial and specialized sectors of the medieval economy hardest [18]. The Black Death devastated medieval Europe, having profound impacts on its socio-economic development, culture, art, religion, and politics [20].

1.3 Cholera

Cholera is an acute, often fatal gastrointestinal disease caused by Vibrio cholerae [21]. Cholera was the first new pandemic threat to the industrial world [15]. Humans become infected through contaminated water used for drinking or food preparation. Historically, seven cholera pandemics have been recognized. Given that India was the place of origin, it is not surprising that cholera mortality there is higher than anywhere else in the world [15]. Subsequently, the spread of cholera was significantly influenced by the transportation revolution: railways and steamships served not only humans but also pathogens [22]. A study [23] estimated that between 1817 and 1860, cholera outbreaks in India caused over 15 million deaths. An additional 23 million people died between 1865 and 1917 during three subsequent outbreaks. The seventh cholera pandemic has severely affected Africa, although the origin and continental spread of the disease have yet to be clearly defined [24]. Table 1 provides information on all seven cholera pandemics.

Table 1 Seven cholera pandemics

Pandemic number	Start year	End year	Estimated deaths	Region(s) affected
1	1817	1824	Unknown	Originated in Bengal, spread through trade routes
2	1829	1837	100,000+	Reached Russia, central Europe, and North America
3	1846	1860	1 million+	John Snow linked cholera to contaminated water
4	1863	1875	600,000+	Spread extensively due to the pilgrimage to Mecca
5	1881	1896	800,000+	Widespread in Europe and South America
6	1899	1923	800,000+	The last serious European outbreak; caused by the El Tor strain
7	1961	Ongoing	Millions	Originated in Indonesia, caused by the El Tor strain

1.4 COVID-19

In December 2019, an outbreak of pneumonia of unknown origin was reported in Wuhan, China. The COVID-19 pandemic has inflicted unprecedented damage on the global economy in terms of human casualties and economic consequences [25]. Thousands of deaths caused by the coronavirus disease prompted the World Health Organization to declare a pandemic on March 12, 2020 [26]. The COVID-19 pandemic has created the largest disruption to educational systems in human history, affecting nearly 1.6 billion students in over 200 countries [27]. The academic performance levels of students are likely to decrease for classes that hold both year-end exams and internal exams, due to reduced contact hours with learners and the lack of consultation with teachers when facing learning/comprehension difficulties [28]. In addition to education, a study [29] claimed that the pandemic affects the economy through the following channels: (1) the direct effect of reduced employment, (2) increased costs of international transactions, (3) a sharp decline in travel, and (4) reduced demand for services requiring close human proximity. COVID-19 negatively impacted the stock market in the form of uncertainty and reduced stock returns worldwide, resulting in decreased capital flows [25]. The damages are not limited to the pandemic period alone. An assessment of the outcomes of implementing an individual rehabilitation plan aimed at lung recovery post-COVID-19 showed that improvement in clinical status and quality of life is mainly dependent on physical performance indicators [30]. The results of a study [31] indicate that the COVID-19 pandemic has affected the mental health of children and young people. These impacts are due to factors such as social isolation from school closures, parental stress about the virus and employment, increased unknown child abuse, increased cyberbullying due to more online activities, and trauma from the loss of family members [32].

Therefore, pandemics pose significant global challenges, causing human casualties, and economic disruptions, and putting pressure on healthcare systems. Traditional methods of prediction and management often fall short when dealing with rapidly spreading diseases. However, advances in generative artificial intelligence offer new ways to detect and predict outbreaks early. This advanced technology can simulate potential pandemic scenarios and enable better preparedness and response strategies. The use of generative artificial intelligence in pandemic prediction has the potential to transform our ability to mitigate the destructive effects of future pandemics. For example, Fig. 1 depicts key elements in the management and prediction of a pandemic.

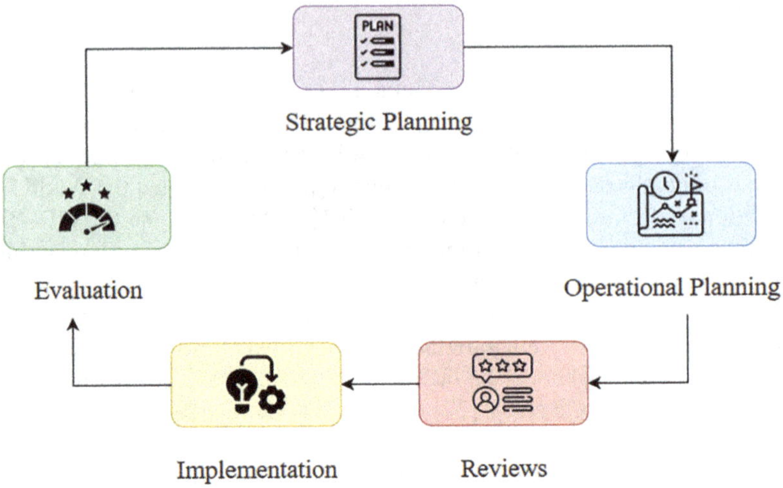

Fig. 1 Key elements in the management and prediction of pandemics

2 Generative AI

Recent advancements in AI have enabled new paradigms of machine processing, shifting from data-driven and discriminatory tasks to complex and creative ones through generative AI [33]. Generative AI is applied in various methods, including text, image, video, code, sound, and other generated content, such as molecules or 3D reconstructions [33]. Generative AI proves to be a catalyst for change across different industries, with healthcare being no exception [34]. In the field of pandemic prediction, generative AI has created new opportunities while also facing challenges that need to be addressed. With advancements in deep learning (DL) techniques, deep generative models have emerged as a class of DL models that generate new content based on existing data, creating new possibilities for AI applications [35]. Consequently, the shift from discriminative to generative AI applications leads to unique use cases and promising opportunities in various fields, including those traditionally resistant to automation [33].

In the field of medicine, particularly in pandemic prediction, generative AI models can be used to simulate various scenarios, analyze the genetic data of viruses, and even generate hypothetical data for modeling disease spread. One of the key factors in accurate pandemic prediction is access to comprehensive and high-quality data. Generative AI can be effective in producing synthetic data from incomplete or limited datasets. For example, by analyzing limited genetic data from viruses, new data can be generated that provides a better understanding of potential virus mutation pathways. Given recent pandemics like COVID-19, the need for more accurate and advanced predictive tools is felt more than ever. Generative AI can serve as one of the critical tools in predicting and managing future pandemics. These models can also assist policymakers at various levels in making better preparations to tackle

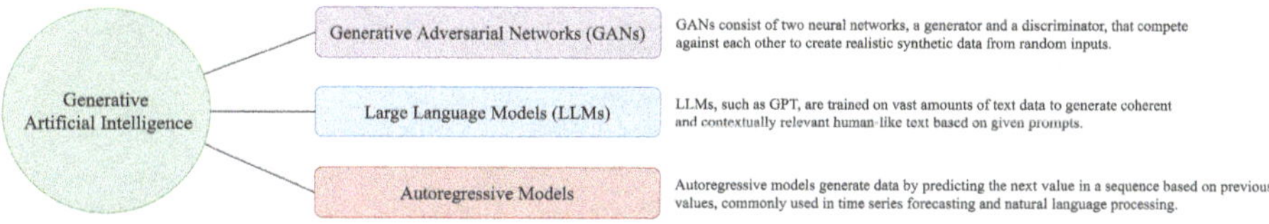

Fig. 2 Types of generative AI

similar crises. In the discussion of generative AI, one of its unique capabilities is the ability to perform unsupervised learning, meaning it can learn from data without explicit labels [34]. Additionally, unlike predictive AI, which uses historical data to forecast future events, generative AI can maintain a "contextual window," leveraging extensive pre-training datasets and incorporating human feedback to guide its algorithms [36]. Gartner has identified five prominent applications of generative AI that are rapidly advancing and finding applications across various industries, including drug design, chip design, materials science, synthetic data generation, and manufacturing parts design [37]. Next, we will introduce three popular generative AI models in the field of pandemic prediction: generative adversarial networks, large language models, and variational auto-encoders. Figure 2 provides an overview of these three categories of generative AI.

2.1 Generative Adversarial Networks

Since their introduction in 2014 [38], GANs have provided a pathway for learning deep representations without extensive training data [39]. The goal of a generative model is to study a set of training examples and learn the probability distribution that created them [40]. In February 2018, GANs achieved a leading position in the list of top ten global technologies published by the Massachusetts Institute of Technology Review [41]. Due to their vast potential for applications including image computation and visualization, speech and language processing, etc., GANs have been widely studied [42]. While common generative models based on deep learning exist, GANs stand out among the most successful generative models (especially in their ability to generate high-resolution, realistic images) [40]. Figure 3 depicts a flowchart of a basic GAN model.

In the study [43], GAN operates based on three principles:

1. Learning a generative model, as well as generating data using certain probabilistic representations.
2. Training a model can be performed under adversarial conditions.

Using deep neural networks and artificial intelligence algorithms to train the complete system [44]. The primary idea behind deploying GAN networks is for unsupervised ML techniques, but it has also been proven to offer better solutions for semi-supervised and reinforcement learning [44].

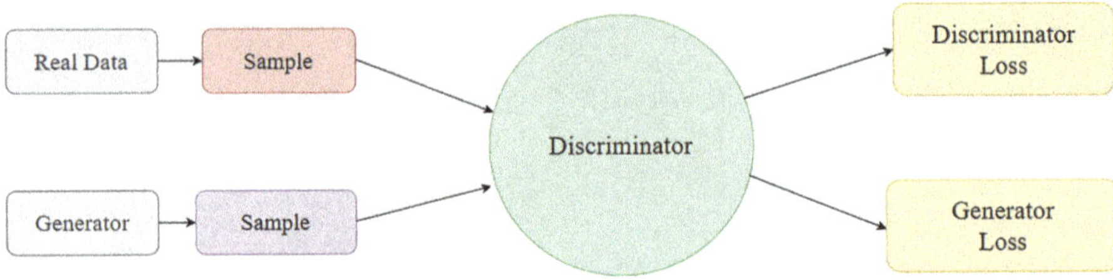

Fig. 3 Flowchart of the basic GAN model

The operation principle of GANs essentially involves training a pair of deep neural networks in competition with each other [39]. GANs consist of two neural networks, a generator and a discriminator, where the generator creates synthetic data. The discriminator is then trained to distinguish between real and synthetic samples. In the dynamic landscape of medicine, GANs have emerged as a transformative technology with manifold advantages [41]. GANs assist in generating specific medical images of individual patients and enable healthcare providers to tailor treatment plans based on patient-specific features [45]. In this section, we aim to highlight the impact of GANs in the prediction and management of pandemics.

2.1.1 Integrating Epidemiology and Deep Learning

In pandemic prediction, the fusion of epidemiology and deep learning has become a powerful approach for enhancing prediction accuracy and providing actionable insights. Traditional epidemiological models, like SEIR (Susceptible, Exposed, Infectious, and Recovered), have limitations when it comes to capturing the complexity of real-world disease spread, especially with evolving factors such as mutation rates and human behavior. Deep learning models, on the other hand, can analyze large datasets and learn from patterns in data without explicit programming. Integrating epidemiological principles with deep learning techniques allows for the modeling of both structured and unstructured data, leading to more accurate and timely pandemic predictions. This approach can support public health authorities by offering real-time insights into disease dynamics, contributing to more effective containment strategies and policy-making during pandemics. Epidemiological prediction during a pandemic is crucial for aiding precise and rapid decision-making (such as various quarantine strategies) by the government to prevent the collapse of the entire medical system [46]. In the study by Wang et al. [46] the T-SIRGAN model is proposed, which integrates the strengths of epidemiological theories and deep learning models to represent complex epidemic processes and model the nonlinear relationship for more accurate COVID-19 growth predictions. T-SIRGAN first uses the Susceptible-Infectious-Recovered (SIR) model to generate epidemiologically-based simulated data, which then serves as adversarial samples for data augmentation in a Generative Adversarial Network (GAN). Transformers are then used to predict future trends of COVID-19 based on the generated synthetic data. The dataset used in this study is from the COVID-19 data repository at Johns Hopkins University. T-SIRGAN consists of three modules: (1) Epidemiological simulation using the SIR model. (2) Data augmentation using GAN. (3) COVID-19 prediction based on Transformers. The proposed T-SIRGAN model first applies epidemiological simulations from the SIR models as adversarial data in GANs, then uses Transformer architecture to predict future COVID-19 trends. Additionally, this model also predicts the COVID-19 epidemic trend assuming no vaccine.

2.1.2 Conditional GAN for Time-Series COVID-19 Predictions

Conditional GANs have proven to be effective for generating realistic data based on conditional inputs. In the context of COVID-19 predictions, conditional GANs can be employed to model and generate time-series data that forecasts the future spread of the virus based on existing data points such as infection rates, mobility data, and healthcare capacity. Unlike traditional statistical models, conditional GANs can adapt to new patterns that emerge in the data, making them ideal for handling non-linear dynamics in pandemic evolution. This approach allows for fine-tuning predictions under different conditions, such as varying social distancing measures or vaccine distribution rates, giving policymakers valuable insights into potential future scenarios. The adaptability of conditional GANs helps in dealing with uncertainties during pandemics. Since COVID-19 cases are essentially time series data, predicting future data is highly necessary [47]. In another study, Bej et al. [47] implemented Conditional GAN (CGAN) to predict future COVID-19 cases in five countries. CGAN, a type of GAN, is used to model and predict COVID-19 cases for the next 3 months with minimal error for the provided dataset. This study uses real WHO-COVID-19 data obtained from https://covid19.who. The authors used 80% of the data as the training dataset and 20% as the testing dataset. This study employed DNN for CGAN, using a six-layer network for the generator section. A three-layer multilayer perceptron receives input x and noise z. On the other hand, the output images are chained to a three-layer network. CGAN captures very complex conditional distributions, whereas various regression methods require different modifications. The predicted and reported data of new COVID cases in India, Italy, Germany, Spain, and the USA from June 6, 2021, to June 10, 2021, show that the reported and predicted data are very close to each other. Therefore, using this model, the economic losses of countries at the end of COVID-19 can be assessed, and preventive measures can be taken to overcome them, helping countries return to normal conditions.

2.1.3 GAN and LSTM Integration for Epidemic Trend Prediction

Integrating GANs with Long Short-Term Memory (LSTM) networks provides a robust framework for predicting epidemic trends. While GANs generate synthetic data that resembles real-time patterns, LSTMs specialize in capturing temporal dependencies and trends over time. This combination can be particularly useful in pandemic prediction by leveraging LSTM's ability to learn from sequential data, such as daily case counts, and GAN's capacity to generate plausible future scenarios. For instance, during COVID-19, this integration can be used to model and forecast surges in infection rates or predict the impact of interventions such as lockdowns. By learning both temporal patterns and data variations, this hybrid model provides more nuanced predictions of pandemic evolution, assisting in better resource allocation and policy responses. In another study, Wang et al. [48] propose an improved machine learning framework using a Generative Adversarial Network (GAN) and Long Short-Term Memory (LSTM) to predict the potential threat of COVID-19 in countries where it is rapidly spreading. The authors also review the latest epidemiological data on COVID-19 before October 18, 2020, and model the epidemic trend as time series data that can be input into the proposed model for data augmentation and epidemic trend prediction. The proposed model is trained to predict the daily number of cumulative confirmed COVID-19 cases in Italy, the USA, China, Germany, the UK, and worldwide.

2.1.4 Machine Learning Techniques for Pandemic Forecasting and City Simulations

Quilodrán et al. [49] state that while epidemiological models can be computationally expensive, recent advances in machine learning techniques have led to neural networks capable of learning and predicting complex changes while reducing computational costs. In this study, the authors introduce two SEIRS digital twin models applied to an "ideal city." In this context, an "ideal city" refers to a hypothetical model or simulation of a city used for simplicity and greater accuracy in analyses and predictions. This ideal city usually has simpler and more controlled features than a real city to allow for more precise study and examination of various parameters. In other words, an ideal city is not a real city but a simplified representation used for modeling and simulations. In this study, predictions from one digital twin based on a modified bidirectional long short-term memory (BDLSTM) network are compared with predictions from another digital twin based on a Generative Adversarial Network (GAN) predictor. The predictions provided by these two frameworks are accurate when compared to the original SEIRS model data and are consistent with each other. Overall, this study proposes a novel reduced-order non-intrusive model (NIROM) based on a bidirectional long short-term memory (BDLSTM) network with a data correction stage derived from BLUE for improved accuracy.

In another study [50] a comparative analysis of three growth curve fitting models (Gompertz, Logistic, and Exponential), two mathematical models (SEIR and IDEA), two forecasting models (Holt Exponential and ARIMA), and four machine/deep learning models (Neural Networks, LSTM networks, GANs, and Random Forest) is presented using three evaluation metrics across ten prominent regions worldwide from North America, South America, Europe, and Asia. The minimum and median values for RMSE were 1.8 and 5372.9, respectively. The mean absolute percentage error values were 0.005 and 6.63, respectively. The AIC values were 87.07 and 613.3 out of a total of 125 experiments in 10 regions. Growth curve fitting models perform well where case smoothing has started. Based on the growth curve of the region, a relevant model from the list can be used to predict the number of COVID-19-infected cases.

2.2 *Large Language Models*

As a primary approach, language modeling has been extensively studied over the past two decades to understand and generate language, evolving from statistical language models to neural language models [51]. Large language models (LLMs) are gaining increasing popularity in academia and industry due to their unprecedented performance across various applications [52]. Recent research on LLMs by academia and industry has advanced significantly, with a notable development being the launch of Chat-GPT, which has garnered widespread attention from the community [51]. Language models can appear remarkably intelligent. This is especially true in extracting correct answers from documents, as they excel in this process due to their mastery of human language and the precise settings they have received in question-and-answer datasets. This process resembles a human agent reading documents to extract information but operates at a much faster rate than a human agent. Large language models leverage numerous elements and processes for their operation. For instance, deep neural networks are a core element in the structure of large language models. These networks aggregate and process linguistic information through a large number of layers and transition pathways. Additionally, large language models benefit from transfer learning; that is, they are initially trained on large text corpora, and subsequently, this knowledge is transferred to smaller models through the weighting of words and sentences. However, it is important to emphasize that such technologies in their current form have the potential to cause harm, an effect well-documented in the field of mental health, where natural language processing algorithms have exhibited biases related to religion, race, and gender [53].

Recognized language models such as Open AI's GPT-4 [54], Anthropic's Claude [55], and Google's PaLM2 [56] have significantly advanced not only the field of artificial intelligence but also the domain of health and medicine. LLMs can assist in generating medical reports or pre-authorization letters based on keywords [57]. Additionally, the study [58] indicates that electronic health records (EHRs), including clinical notes, are among the largest, fastest-growing, and most data-rich sources available. This is partly due to the lack of interoperability and standardization—syntactic, structural, and semantic—hindering efficient interpretation and knowledge retrieval. LLMs can help overcome these barriers. Furthermore, the Alpha-Fold system by DeepMind, which is associated with one of the most exciting advancements in artificial intelligence of our time, is capable of predicting the structure and thus

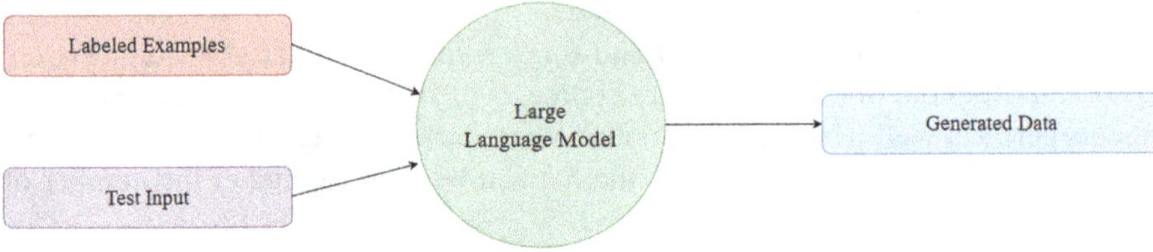

Fig. 4 A Flowchart of large language models

the biological function of nearly any protein. Figure 4 illustrates a flowchart of how LLMs operate.

It should be noted that LLMs connect responses together without inherently being able to show the logic behind their work. This task is delegated to the human operator, who can only perform reliably if the model provides insights into its data sources and labels the AI-generated content accordingly [58]. In healthcare, LLMs might be classified into LLMs for biomedical fields and LLMs for clinical fields based on the bodies of text used for pre-training classification [59]. Additionally, new architectures, such as the Hybrid Value-Aware Transformer (HVAT), may further enhance the performance of LLMs by allowing for the integration of longitudinal and multifaceted clinical data [60]. Next, we will identify studies that have performed best in the field of pandemic prediction.

2.2.1 LLM-Based Framework for Social Media Analysis in Public Health

LLMs such as GPT-4 can be highly effective in public health by analyzing vast amounts of social media data. During a pandemic, people often turn to platforms like Twitter and Facebook to share information, ask questions, or express concerns. An LLM-based framework can analyze this data to identify trends such as rising anxiety about a particular health issue, misinformation about treatments, or emerging symptoms reported by the public. This real-time data extraction allows public health authorities to gauge the public's mood, spot potential outbreaks, or intervene in cases of widespread misinformation. By integrating LLMs with existing surveillance systems, it becomes possible to create an early-warning system that detects and responds to public health issues through the lens of social media sentiment. In the study by Ding et al. [61], a multi-stage reasoning framework using LLMs is introduced to examine the relationship between social media patterns and trends in national health outcomes. Based on the theory of fuzzy tracking, which emphasizes the importance of "topics" of causal coherence ineffective health communications, the authors introduce Role-Based Incremental Coaching (RBIC), a real-time LLM-based framework for large-scale event detection. Using RBIC, key points from subreddit discussions opposing COVID-19 health measures can be systematically extracted. The authors identified the most prominent clusters, covering the main topics at the heart of how and why people opposed public health measures across

COVID-19, from May 2020 to October 2021. A total of 79,680 posts were collected from subreddits between May 2020 and October 2021 [61]:

> conspiracy commons, Coronavirus Circle jerk, Coronavirus FOS, Coronavirus Rights, COVID-19, covid-19 testimonials, covid vaccinated uncut, Vax Kampf, Debate Vaccines, Fauci For Prison, ivermectin, lock down skepticism, No New Normal, true anti-vaccination, vaccine long haulers, VAERS reports, Wuhan Flu, Covid Is A Fraud, COVID-19 Origin, church of covid.

The authors implemented S-BERT using Sentence Transformer to extract embedding from its core. The S-BERT model consists of 12 hidden layers, each generating an output representation of specific dimensions. To obtain high-quality embedding, output representations were extracted from each of the last three hidden layers of the model (layers 10–12) and averaged. While this focus allows for in-depth analysis of the main posts, it may not encompass the complete discourse, including diverse viewpoints and nuanced discussions that often occur in the comments section [61].

2.2.2 LLM Integration in Multi-modal Medical Models for COVID-19

During pandemics like COVID-19, multi-modal medical models that combine various data sources—such as patient symptoms, imaging, and genetic information—are vital for comprehensive disease prediction and management. By incorporating Large Language Models (LLMs), which can process and interpret complex textual data, into these multi-modal systems, we enhance the ability to analyze electronic health records, patient narratives, and research literature. LLMs can draw connections between diverse medical inputs and current research to support clinical decision-making. This integration proves valuable in improving the diagnosis, treatment recommendations, and even the prediction of long-term effects in COVID-19 patients. With LLMs, the predictive models can synthesize complex datasets more efficiently, helping healthcare providers respond to pandemics with greater precision and speed. In another study by Liu et al. [62] a multi-modal medical large language model (Med-MLLM) was reported for learning radiographic representations, which can acquire extensive medical knowledge (e.g., image understanding, text semantics, and clinical phenotypes) from unlabeled data. Consequently, when faced with a rare disease, Med-MLLM can quickly adapt and easily adjust to limited labels. Additionally, the proposed model supports medical data across visual modalities (e.g., chest X-rays and CT scans) and textual methods (e.g., medical reports and free-text clinical notes). Therefore, it can be used for clinical tasks involving both visual and textual data. Experiments are conducted on (1) three types of input data; (2) three types of downstream tasks including disease reporting, diagnosis, and prognosis; (3) five COVID-19 datasets; and (4) three different languages including English, Chinese, and Spanish. All experiments show that the proposed model can support accurate and robust decision-making for COVID-19 with limited labeled data. The authors used an image encoder and an additional text decoder for fine-tuning (cross-entropy optimization) the pre-trained Med-MLLM on COVID-19 reporting tasks (medical report generation). For the COVID-19 diagnosis task (disease classification), a classification layer is added to the output of image and/or text encoders, and Med-MLLM is fine-tuned using binary cross-entropy loss. For the COVID-19 prognosis task (survival prediction), the authors adopted the same fine-tuning strategy as for the COVID-19 diagnosis task, as the two tasks differ only in the output results. Both tasks can accept three types of medical input data: image-only, text-only, and image-text. Finally, the authors evaluated the performance of their framework on five COVID-19 datasets across different methods, languages, and regions, including the COVIDx-CXR-2 dataset, the COVID-CXR dataset, the COVID-19 CT dataset, the BIMCV-COVID-19 dataset, and the COVID-HCH dataset. It should be noted that despite the model's good performance compared to traditional models, this approach does not perform well for the Omicron variant.

2.2.3 Developing Multi-modal Predictive Models in Pandemic Prediction

Multi-modal predictive models leverage a combination of various data types—such as clinical, genomic, environmental, and social media data—to provide a more holistic approach to pandemic prediction. In contrast to uni-modal models that only focus on a single data source, multi-modal models can capture a richer set of features, improving predictive accuracy. For example, during COVID-19, integrating data from medical records, mobility patterns, and real-time infection data offers a more comprehensive understanding of how the virus spreads and mutates. By using AI models such as GANs and LLMs to fuse these diverse data types, predictive models can anticipate new hotspots, forecast healthcare needs, and suggest tailored intervention strategies. This multi-modal approach is critical for managing future pandemics, enabling quicker and more informed decision-making. In another study, Agarwal et al. [63] proposed a transfer learning approach using COVID-19 as a case study to develop predictive models from multi-modal electronic health records by leveraging information from more common diseases with shared clinical features. The new hierarchical and multi-modal model integrates baseline risk factors from natural language processing of clinical notes at admission, time-series measurements of biomarkers obtained from laboratory tests, and discrete diagnostic, procedural, and medication codes. Compared to clinical observations like diagnostic codes, procedures, and laboratory tests that typically indicate the onset of a problem, medication duration allows us to reason about the type and severity of a specific symptom and its short-term and long-term impact. The authors' experiments show that their hierarchical transfer learning approach, using severe respiratory disease (SRD) groups, results in improvements of 12.9 and 10.3% in AUROC for predicting COVID-19 patient stay and ventilation. The authors evaluate their implementation with three models representing distinct predictive approaches, demonstrating improvements between 5.8–29.2% in AUROC and 3.6–66% in F1 score for ventilation prediction tasks. This approach accurately predicts the short-term and long-term probability of a patient's condition. Using STARR OMOP data, the authors created a cohort of COVID-19 patients based on study entry criteria: (1) patients visited after January 1, 2020, (2) patients older than 18 years at admission, (3) patients who either had a positive COVID-19 test within 14 days before admission or were diagnosed with COVID-19 within 7 days before admission.

The study by Yang et al. [65] introduces Pandemic-LLM, a new framework using multi-modal large language models (LLM) that reformulates real-time disease outbreak prediction as a textual reasoning problem, with the ability to integrate real-time, complex, and non-numeric information. This approach encodes multi-modal data for LLMs through a rapid collaboration design with unique artificial intelligence and time series representation learning. Empirically, Pandemic-LLM has demonstrated itself to be a high-performance pandemic prediction framework that effectively shows the impact of emerging variants and can provide timely and accurate predictions. An extensive evaluation of Pandemic-LLM across 50 U.S. states over 16 weeks highlights its benefits: Pandemic-LLM offers strong and reliable predictions and delivers classified predictions with confidence levels that support public health policymaking. Additionally, it shows timely and accurate responses to emerging pandemic types and utilizes timely genomic surveillance data analysis. These findings showcase the potential use of LLMs in public health emergency response settings. Specifically, Pandemic-LLM integrates real-time textual virology features, estimated variant prevalence, public health policy text, and healthcare system performance with traditional demographic and epidemiological time series. The inclusion of variable information has been shown to enhance model performance without the need for retraining, emphasizing the importance of adapting to real-time information for effective responses during ongoing outbreaks. In summary, the goal of the rapid AI-human collaboration design is to enable real-time automation and allow human expertise to strategically focus on selecting the most relevant and timely information from trusted sources, such as updated policies and various reports.

2.2.4 LLM for Unsupervised Learning in Medical Imaging and Text Analysis

LLMs are commonly used in natural language processing, but their capabilities extend to unsupervised learning tasks in both medical imaging and text analysis. In the realm of medical imaging, LLMs can process textual reports, extracting meaningful insights and correlations between text data and image findings. This is particularly valuable for tasks like radiology report generation or identifying abnormalities that correlate with specific symptoms. In an unsupervised learning context, LLMs can analyze vast amounts of unlabeled medical data, identifying hidden patterns that might not be immediately apparent. For instance, LLMs can cluster similar medical cases or imaging results without the need for explicit labels, uncovering new disease subtypes or identifying novel relationships between patient history and diagnostic imaging. Combining text and imaging data through LLMs accelerates the discovery of new medical insights, which can be invaluable during pandemics when large-scale data is abundant but labeled data is scarce. In another study, Liu et al. [64] proposed a multi-modal large language model—Unsupervised Learning from Medical Images and Text (ULUMIT)—for learning radiographic representations, which can acquire extensive medical knowledge (e.g., image understanding, text semantics, and clinical phenotypes) from unlabeled data. Consequently, when faced with a rare disease, the authors' framework can quickly adapt and easily accommodate limited labels. Moreover, ULUMIT supports medical data from all visual modalities (e.g., chest X-rays and CT scans) and textual methods (e.g., medical reports and free-text clinical notes). Therefore, it can be used for clinical tasks involving both visual and textual medical data. Besides COVID-19, the authors' framework can also be applied to identify 14 common chest diseases and tuberculosis across five additional public datasets, demonstrating its robustness in generalization and transferability. For COVID-19 diagnosis (disease classification), a linear layer (e.g., a classification layer) is added to the output of image and/or text encoders. The authors evaluate their framework's performance on five COVID-19 datasets across different methods, languages, and regions, such as COVIDx-CXR-2, COVID-CXR, COVID-19 CT dataset, BIMCV-COVID-19 dataset, and COVID-HCH dataset. The proposed approach achieves promising results without using labeled downstream data for training, whereas previous methods show a significant decrease in performance, with more than a 30% reduction in AUC score.

The study [67] examines the combination of various models based on BERT and CNN used for sentiment analysis in tweets related to COVID-19. The aim of this research is to provide solutions for improving the accuracy of sentiment analysis and to explore the cultural and computational limitations in analyzing social data related to phenomena such as the COVID-19 pandemic. This could play a key role in better managing global health crises. The authors, recognizing the importance of understanding public sentiment in the context of policy-making, crisis management, and public health, strive to offer an efficient and lightweight approach to sentiment analysis through a detailed analysis of these models and by proposing new research directions. This approach, aimed at enhancing methods for predicting and managing pandemics through the analysis of social data and the use of advanced models, plays an important role in rapid and effective decision-making in response to health crises. The authors highlight the weaknesses of CNN-based models, particularly their lack of attention to semantic relationships within texts, which can reduce accuracy. They introduce BERT as a suitable alternative. By leveraging masking methods, BERT reduces the need for complex domain-specific frameworks and delivers outstanding performance across various text-related tasks. The authors also address the challenges of sentiment analysis in informal tweets written during the COVID-19 pandemic and attempt to improve performance in analyzing large and diverse datasets using deep models like BERT and CNN. Emphasizing the need for more comprehensive and multilingual data, the authors point out the current limitations of research, including the focus on English texts and short time periods.

2.2.5 AI-Driven Drug Target Identification for Global Health Threats

AI-driven drug target identification plays a pivotal role in addressing global health threats such as pandemics. The process of identifying drug targets—specific proteins or genes involved in the progression of a disease—can be significantly accelerated using AI models like deep learning and generative algorithms. These models can sift through vast genomic and proteomic datasets, identifying potential targets for drug development far faster than traditional methods. AI can analyze disease mechanisms at a molecular level, revealing potential vulnerabilities in pathogens such as SARS-CoV-2, which causes COVID-19. Moreover, AI-driven approaches can simulate drug-target interactions, predict the efficacy of potential compounds, and propose new drug candidates for clinical trials. During global health crises, rapid identification of drug targets is crucial for developing vaccines, antivirals, or therapeutic interventions, and AI's capacity to handle this complex process at scale ensures a quicker response to emerging threats. The study [66] explores the capabilities of ChatGPT in the rapid identification of drugs in response to global health threats. This research investigates and evaluates an automated framework for analyzing scientific literature related to SARS-CoV-2 and Nipah viruses. The authors introduce an innovative method, aiming to enable the swift identification of drug targets for various viruses by utilizing artificial intelligence and advanced prompt engineering techniques. This approach, which is based on assessing various articles and aligning the performance of the automated system with expert human opinions, plays a crucial role in the rapid detection and prevention of pandemics. The findings demonstrate the effectiveness of ChatGPT in accelerating the drug discovery process during health emergencies, significantly improving the management of crises caused by emerging diseases. In this study, the authors' best configuration, using GPT-4, achieved performance metrics for SARS-CoV-2 with an accuracy of 92.87%, F1-score of 88.43%, sensitivity of 83.38%, and specificity of 97.82%. For Nipah, the metrics were 87.40% for accuracy, 73.90% for F1-score, 74.72% for sensitivity, and 91.36% for specificity. These results indicate that using ChatGPT in drug discovery is highly beneficial and has the potential to aid in the rapid identification of drug targets during health emergencies at a pandemic scale.

2.3 Autoregressive

These models predict the next output in a sequence based on previous outputs. They have been used extensively in language modeling tasks (like text generation), as well as in generating music and even images [68].

2.3.1 Advanced Time Series Models for Epidemic Forecasting

In the study by Hwang et al. [69] the authors adopt heterogeneous autoregressive (HAR) time series models and discussed statistical inference for various COVID-19 data. A HAR model, which is a robust and interesting time series model for structured data with long memory, has recently garnered significant attention from economists and statisticians in time series analysis. Seven datasets, such as cumulative confirmed cases (CC), cumulative recovered cases (CR), and cumulative death cases (CD), as well as recovery rate, mortality rate, and infection rate for 14 and 21 days, are used for statistical analysis. In this work, instead of the traditional ARIMA model, HAR models are used to study the estimation and prediction of Korean COVID-19 time series data. The HAR model with geometrically weighted cosine innovation conditions is an interesting model for fitting the COVID-19 series worldwide or in other countries with similar fluctuating characteristics.

In another study, Rajab et al. [70] proposed an approach for predicting the spread of epidemics based on vector autoregression models. Specifically, the authors combined time series for new cases and new deaths to create a joint forecasting model. They applied the proposed model to predict the number of new cases and deaths in the United Arab Emirates, Saudi Arabia, and Kuwait. Out-of-sample testing results show that the proposed model achieves a high level of accuracy, outperforming many existing methods. Specifically, the proposed approach achieves mean absolute percentage errors (MAPE) of 0.35, 2.03, and 3.75% in predicting daily new case counts for the three countries, respectively. Additionally, with in sample predictions for cumulative case counts, MAPE values of 0.0017, 0.002, and 0.024% are obtained, respectively. The data used in this study includes daily counts of new cases and deaths collected for the three countries. To obtain a more balanced and suitable time series, the authors utilized a 7-day moving average. While taking the first difference stabilized the series around zero, additional transformations could be used to improve variance. This model could be beneficial with further expansion and inclusion of variables such as tested population percentages, recovered cases, and other factors.

In another study, Sioofy et al. [71] proposed a network autoregressive (NAR) model to predict the total number of COVID-19 cases in Iran by the end of December 2021, taking into account the disease interactions in neighboring countries. To this end, COVID-19 data were initially collected for seven countries in the region, including Iran, Turkey, Iraq, Azerbaijan, Armenia, Afghanistan, and Pakistan. A network was then created for these countries, and the correlation of disease data was calculated. After introducing the main structure of the NAR model, a mathematical framework was subsequently provided to further integrate the correlation matrix into the prediction process. Additionally, maximum likelihood estimation (MLE) was used to determine the model parameters and optimize prediction accuracy. By incorporating the correlation matrix into the NAR model, which was designed to observe the disease's cross-impact on neighboring countries, the number of infected cases in Iran was predicted for December 2021. Furthermore, an integrated autoregressive moving average (ARIMA) model was used as a benchmark to compare and validate the results of the NAR model. Combining disease interactions not only aids the algorithm but also evaluates one of the most significant components of disease transmission between communities, significantly enhancing the accuracy of time series predictions. This is examined by comparing the ARIMA and NARI models. The RMSE values with and without considering disease interactions in neighboring countries are 5.42 and 3.06 for ARIMA and NARI, respectively. This indicates that accounting for disease interactions in neighboring countries significantly improves prediction accuracy. As the model's accuracy in predicting disease increases, more reliable tools are provided for policymakers to make informed control decisions.

2.3.2 Dynamic Forecasting of COVID-19 Cases Using ARIMA Models

AutoRegressive Integrated Moving Average (ARIMA) models are widely used for time-series forecasting due to their ability to capture trends, seasonality, and noise in data. In the context of pandemic prediction, ARIMA models have proven useful for dynamically forecasting COVID-19 case numbers by analyzing historical data on infection rates, deaths, and recoveries. ARIMA models work well in situations where past data can inform future trends, making them suitable for short-term predictions during the early and peak phases of an outbreak. By continuously updating the model with real-time data, ARIMA can adapt to changing patterns, such as the effect of lockdowns or vaccination campaigns on the spread of the virus. However, ARIMA models are most effective when combined with more advanced AI techniques like deep learning, which can handle non-linearities and complex dependencies that ARIMA models may miss. Together, these methods can provide robust forecasts that guide public health interventions and resource allocation during pandemics. In another study, Melin et al. [72] analyzed dynamic models to generate 20-day forecasts of cumulative confirmed deaths and recoveries from COVID-19 based on country, territory, or transportation data produced on April 24, 2020. The United States, Spain, Italy, France, Germany, the United Kingdom, Turkey, Iran, China, Russia, Brazil, Canada, Belgium, the Netherlands, and Switzerland were selected based on cumulative effect data from the top 20 countries. In the ARIMA model, a weight was assigned to past values, and an error term was allocated for model correction. The authors collected case data for each day at specified times from January 21, 2020, to April 24, 2020. Additionally, data from the top 15 countries, along with their geographical locations, were preprocessed to create spatial features. Daily COVID-19 data were collected and cumulatively displayed as a spatial map for over 170 countries and regions. The spatial map was useful for identifying the severity of COVID-19 infections in the top 15 countries and continents. Recent reported data for confirmed cases, deaths, and recoveries over the past 3 months (from January to April 2020) were presented and compared among the top 15 infected countries. The ARIMA model was used to forecast confirmed cases, deaths, and recoveries in the top 15 countries from April 24 to July 7, 2020. The model's results were shown with 95, 80, and 70% confidence intervals. Confidence intervals were displayed as the average range between 80 and 70%. The ARIMA model's validation was performed using AIC for the available recent data, with values approximately 20, 14, and 16 for cumulative confirmed cases, deaths, and recoveries from COVID-19, respectively, indicating acceptable results. Observed predicted values suggest that confirmed cases, deaths, and recoveries in all countries except China, Switzerland, and Germany would double. The accuracy of the country data collected from Worldometer for the entire study was deemed reliable.

The use of generative artificial intelligence in epidemic forecasting offers a transformative approach to understanding and managing health crises. GANs, LLMs, and autoregressive models each play a unique role in this field. GANs can simulate diverse scenarios, LLMs provide insightful analysis from extensive datasets, and autoregressive models accurately predict future trends. Integrating these technologies enhances our forecasting capabilities, leading to more effective and timely responses to pandemics, ultimately saving lives and resources.

3 Advantages of Using Generative AI for Pandemic Prediction

Using generative AI in epidemic prediction offers significant advantages. These techniques, with their ability to simulate and analyze complex data, can reveal hidden patterns and provide accurate predictions of disease spread. Additionally, generative AI can rapidly simulate various scenarios, providing policymakers and researchers with powerful tools for timely and effective decision-making. These approaches have several advantages over traditional methods, which are detailed below.

3.1 Traditional Models

These models, such as Susceptible-Infected-Recovered (SIR) and Susceptible-Exposed-Infected-Recovered (SEIR), divide the population into compartments based on disease status. Transitions between compartments are described using differential equations, allowing the simulation of disease dynamics over time.

3.1.1 SIR

The study [73] states that one way to model the spread of infectious diseases is by dividing the affected population into different compartments. In the Susceptible-Infected-Recovered (SIR) model, the entire population is categorized into susceptible, infected, and recovered sections. This model assumes that recovered individuals cannot be re-infected. The SEIR model adds an additional "Exposed" compartment for individuals who have been infected but are not yet infectious after an incubation period. The models are deterministic and move from left to right: a susceptible person may move to the exposed compartment, an exposed person to the infected compartment, and an infected person to the recovered compartment. These models form the basis for many more complex models that include geography, multiple age groups, and other factors.

The SIR model was first introduced by Kermack and McKendrick in 1927 [74]. They successfully used it to model an epidemic on the island of Bombay in 1905–1906. Since then, numerous studies on the SIR model and its applications, both on its own and as part of more complex models, have been conducted [73]. The SIR model is considered one of the simplest types of dynamic models, and many other types of models are derived from this basic model. The SIR model is capable of predicting contagious diseases that are transmitted from person to person, where recovered individuals become resistant to reinfection. This model has been used for almost a century to study the plague. Significant advancements in studying dynamic epidemics were made in the mid-twentieth century. In recent decades, various influential factors have been added to the classic SIR model [75]. Designing an SIR model for an epidemic disease requires determining several key parameters such as the infection rate and the removal rate, either empirically or statistically. Using more complex models with greater accuracy and detail requires extensive and accurate data. This model is a dynamic system described by three equations that outline the temporal changes of three populations:

1. Susceptible Individuals S(t): This group consists of individuals who are not currently infected but may become infected. These individuals might either become infected or remain susceptible.
2. Infected Individuals I(t): This group comprises individuals who have been infected with the virus and can transmit it to susceptible individuals. An infected person may either be re-infected, recover, or die.
3. Removed Individuals R(t): This group includes individuals who have either recovered or died. Additionally, it is assumed that the time scale of the SIR model is such that births and deaths unrelated to the virus can be ignored.

Furthermore, a study [76] proposes an SIR-based framework, which is an integrated model that encompasses multiple waves of daily reported cases. The existing epidemic growth function models are shown as specific cases of the GSIR model. Dynamic parameter modeling reflects the impact of policy decisions, social awareness, and the availability of medication during the pandemic. The GSIR framework can be used to find an appropriate or predictive model for any epidemic. This study was conducted on COVID-19 data for various countries, with accurate results for India, Brazil, the United States (USA), and the world. Peak infections, the total expected number of COVID-19 cases and deaths, the time-varying reproductive number, and various other parameters are estimated from available data using the proposed method. The proposed GSIR model enhances existing theory and provides promising results for continuous predictive monitoring of the COVID-19 pandemic. The parameters of the SIR model include:

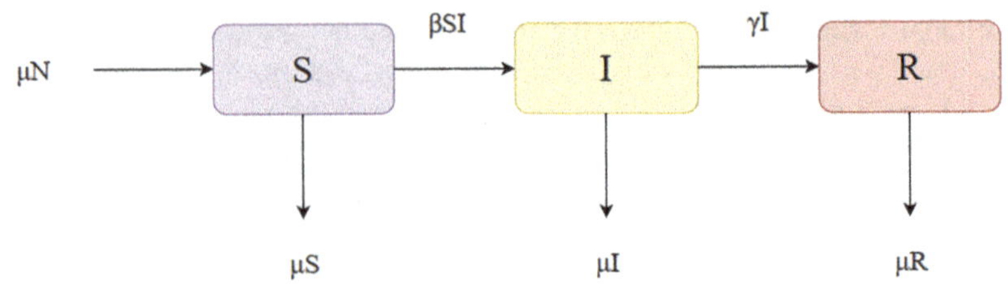

Fig. 5 Traditional model steps of the SIR model

- β (Beta)—Transmission Rate: This is the probability of disease transmission from an infected individual to a susceptible individual during each encounter. This parameter indicates the intensity and speed of disease spread in the community.
- γ (Gamma)—Recovery Rate: The rate at which infected patients recover and transition to the recovered category. This parameter is defined as the inverse of the average duration of the disease.
- μ (Mu)—Natural Mortality Rate: This parameter represents the natural mortality rate or the rate of exit from the population due to reasons other than the disease being studied. It is usually expressed as a daily or weekly rate and allows the model to account for the impact of natural mortality, leading to greater accuracy.

Figure 5 summarizes the steps of the SEIR approach.

3.1.2 SEIR

The SEIR structure is an extension of the SIR structure. In other words, this approach includes an additional compartment called "E" for exposed individuals who have been infected by the virus but are not yet infectious, in addition to the S, I, and R compartments [74]. In many cases, there are no visible symptoms infected individuals such as chicken pox, tuberculosis etc. and in that cases an SEIR model is mostly used [77]. The spread of infection starts with the introduction of a small group of infected individuals into a larger population. Then the population (N) is divided into four classes: Susceptible (S), Exposed (E), Infected (I), and Recovered (R) at any time $t \geq 0$ [78]. The study [79] states that generally, the traditional SEIR model (Susceptible-Exposed-Infected-Recovered) is used to describe the spread of viruses with an incubation period. For the COVID-19 pandemic, the SEIR model has been improved based on the following analysis:

With the increased capability of nucleic acid detection, E no longer represents the size of the virus carrier group in the incubation period, but rather the size of virus carriers with a low viral load that is not detectable. Similarly, I represent the size of virus carriers that can be detected [79].

- Considering isolation measures during the COVID-19 epidemic, a new class Q is added to describe the size of the currently isolated group [79].

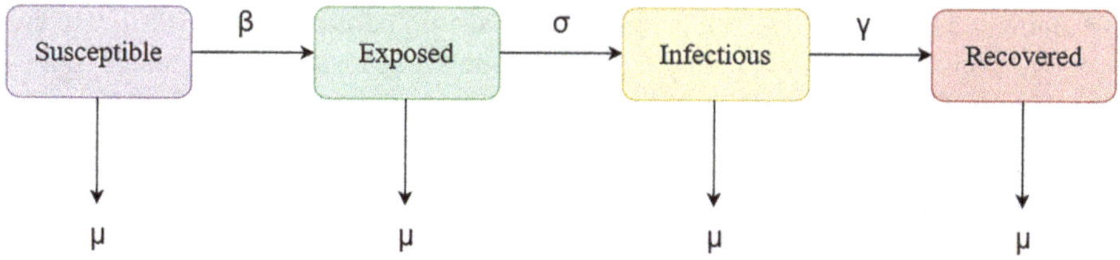

Fig. 6 Traditional model steps of the SEIR model

- The size of temporarily removed individuals is represented by R. This refers to the group size that has temporary immunity or is not exposed to the environment due to protective measures. Such considerations can describe not only the secondary infection of recovered individuals due to virus mutation but also the protective measures for susceptible individuals [79].

In general, it can be said that mathematical modeling is an efficient method if the parameters can be accurately estimated. The parameters of the SIR model include the following:

- **β (Beta)**—Transmission rate: Equal to the probability of disease transmission from an infected individual to a susceptible individual during each encounter. This parameter indicates the intensity and speed of disease spread in the community.
- **γ (Gamma)**—Recovery rate: The rate at which infected patients recover and move to the recovered category. This parameter is defined as the inverse of the average duration of the disease.
- **μ (Mu)**—Natural mortality rate: The parameter "μ" (mu) is defined as the natural mortality rate or the rate of exit from the population (due to reasons other than the disease under study). This parameter is usually expressed as a daily or weekly rate and allows the model to consider the impact of natural mortality on the population for greater accuracy.
- **σ (Sigma)**—Conversion rate from exposed to infected: The rate at which exposed individuals become infected. This parameter is the inverse of the average incubation period of the disease.

Figure 6 summarizes the stages of the SEIR approach.

3.2 Advantages of GAI-Based Models Over Traditional Models

Sections 2.1–2.3 introduced AI-based models that have higher capabilities in analyzing and more accurately predicting the trends of pandemics compared to traditional approaches. These models, using extensive data and complex architectures, can simulate the behavior and spread of diseases more precisely, significantly aiding health decision-making. While traditional methods have been effective in advancing our understanding of disease dynamics, they have numerous limitations. There are many reasons for this discrepancy between models and reality, but we can summarize them as follows:

Data Dependency Traditional models often rely on high-quality and extensive data, which can be challenging to obtain in the early stages of an outbreak or in resource-limited settings. These approaches also tend to perform poorly with very limited data. For example, during the COVID-19 pandemic, the data collection period was short, so a significant proportion of the data was likely inaccurate [80]. On the other hand, generative AI can produce synthetic data that mimics real-world data, which can be used to augment limited datasets and improve model training. This capability is particularly valuable when dealing with sparse or incomplete data. Therefore, the dependence on data in AI-based models is much less than in traditional models.

Assumptions Many traditional models make simplifying assumptions about disease transmission and population behavior that may not accurately reflect real-world complexities. Additionally, most of these models work on a small sample of the discussed population. Also, when a disease is largely known in a population, many of its individuals develop immunity, but the same diseases can devastate whole populations if these diseases are new within these groups (this was the case of measles, smallpox, pertussis, and influenza) [81]. On the other hand, generative AI models can be continuously updated with new data, allowing them to adapt to changing conditions and provide real-time predictions. In this scenario, there are no simplifying assumptions that create a significant gap between reality and model predictions.

Real-Time Decision-Making Traditional models may struggle to adapt quickly to rapidly changing conditions, such as the emergence of new variants or shifts in public behavior. This can limit their effectiveness in real-time decision-making. Conversely, generative AI models can be continuously updated with new data, enabling them to adapt to changing conditions and provide real-time predictions. This ability is crucial for responding to rapidly evolving outbreaks. In general, mathematical models of disease spread are very useful for simulating the behavior of a pandemic if a specific intervention is taken or if there are particular changes in the pathogen or host, assuming other variables remain constant [81].

Scalability Some traditional models, especially agent-based models, can be computationally intensive and challenging to scale for large populations or complex scenarios. In contrast, generative models can learn complex, nonlinear relationships within the data and capture intricate patterns that traditional models might overlook. This capability allows for more precise and accurate predictions. Additionally, generative AI can integrate diverse data sources such as epidemiological data, genomic data, and mobility patterns to create comprehensive predictive models. This holistic approach enhances the accuracy and robustness of predictions. Generative AI can simulate various outbreak scenarios, helping public health authorities assess the potential impacts of different interventions and prepare for worst-case scenarios.

Other Reasons Some obvious reasons include public health interventions such as case detection, border control, regional quarantine, travel restrictions, antiviral treatment and prevention, case isolation, home quarantine, reactive school/workplace closures, promoting remote work, adjusting the capacity of public spaces, social distancing, and vaccination [82]. Although each one of these interventions can be modeled and their effects evaluated under fixed conditions, in reality, the application of these interventions changes over space, time, intensity, and adherence making it very difficult to foresee their real effect [81]. The study [81] states that, generally, mathematical models of the spread of disease are very useful to simulate the behavior of an epidemic if a given intervention is adopted or if there are specific changes in the pathogen or the host, assuming all other variables are kept fixed. They are also useful for understanding the past and tracking an epidemic in real time. However, their predictive power can be rather questionable due to the space-time-biological-societal changing nature of the problem that cannot be forecasted by the model. This was well illustrated in the case of the Ebola outbreak between 2013–2016.

4 Applications of Generative AI in Pandemic Prediction

The use of generative AI in predicting pandemics has wide-ranging applications. This technology can create complex models for simulating and analyzing epidemiological data, aiding in more accurate predictions of disease spread. Additionally, generative AI can simulate various scenarios to evaluate the impacts of health interventions, contributing to better and more effective decision-making in managing health crises. Below are some practical applications and uses in this field:

Real-Time Monitoring Generative AI plays a crucial role in enhancing real-time monitoring systems during pandemics. Learning from previous viruses and creating a rapid response mechanism can be effective in identifying and containing new diseases [83]. By integrating data from various sources, such as health records, social media, and mobility data, generative models can detect early signs of disease outbreaks and monitor their spread in real time. For example, AI-based health systems can analyze social media posts, news articles, user comments, and search engine queries to identify emerging pandemics. These monitoring systems can also generate alerts for authorities and officials, enabling a swift response to contain outbreaks before they escalate.

Resource Allocation and Management Effective resource allocation during a pandemic is crucial to ensure that healthcare facilities are not overwhelmed and that resources are distributed equitably. For instance, when news of the COVID-19 outbreak spread in various countries, there was a surge in the purchase of health items like masks, gloves, and disinfectants, leading to profiteering by some individuals. The shortage of these health items at the city or country level and the public's concern about securing and maintaining health resources raised their voices in protest. This was in a context where alarming news was increasing worldwide, and medical experts, due to the novelty of the disease, offered no definitive cure or even preventive measures. The lack of planning forced policymakers to make ad-hoc decisions about resource acquisition and allocation, which might exacerbate shortages [84]. Although few children required hospitalization due to symptomatic infection, they could still be significantly affected by the strain on the healthcare system imposed by the pandemic and should be considered in resource allocation frameworks [85]. Generative AI can assist in this process by predicting the demand for medical equipment, hospital beds, and healthcare personnel based on current and projected disease trends. AI models can simulate various scenarios and identify and recommend the most efficient solutions for resource distribution.

Disease Spread Forecasting New infections are introduced based on interactions, adherence to distancing norms, hygiene levels, and other social interventions among a susceptible population from an un-quarantined infected population [86]. Generative AI models, such as GANs and Variational Autoencoders (VAEs), are highly effective in forecasting disease spread. These models can simulate different scenarios by learning underlying patterns and structures in epidemiological data. By generating synthetic data that reflects real-world conditions, generative AI can improve the accuracy of predictions and help public health authorities understand how a disease might spread under various circumstances. This capability is especially useful in predicting future infection rates, identifying potential high-risk areas, and planning interventions.

5 Challenges and Limitations

The use of generative AI in predicting pandemics comes with challenges and limitations. These challenges include the need for high-quality, large-volume data, the complexity of models, and heavy computational demands. Additionally, issues related to inaccurate or incomplete data, ethical and privacy concerns, and inherent uncertainties in epidemiological predictions are other obstacles facing this technology.

Model Interpretability Generative AI models are often considered "black boxes" due to their complex architecture. The interpretability of GANs has attracted increasing attention in recent years [87]. As users begin to interact with generative adversarial networks (GANs) more frequently, there is a need for ways to explain the computational system to them so that they know that the GAN generative process is reasonable [88]. This lack of interpretability makes it difficult for public health officials and policymakers to understand how the models arrive at their predictions. The opaque nature of these models can hinder trust and acceptance. Enhancing the interpretability of generative AI models is crucial for building trust and ensuring their effective use in pandemic prediction. Generally, the more complex an architecture is, the more hidden interactions and assumptions remain out of sight for users and developers.

Data Quality and Availability High-quality data are crucial for training generative AI models. However, during pandemics like Ebola, obtaining accurate and large-scale data can be challenging due to factors such as limited data quantity, delays, poor data collection quality, and low confidence in data accuracy across different regions. These limitations can lead to biases in models and significantly affect the accuracy of predictions. If the collected data for training the model is incomplete, of low quality, or contains errors, the generative AI model may produce unreliable predictions, impacting decision-making processes. The more data is publicly available the more transparency, accountability, and democratization of the research process is enabled, allowing a sound evidence-based analysis of the consequences of health policies [89]. Table 2 shows a list of up-to-date data sources for each country during the COVID-19 pandemic.

Ethical and Privacy Concerns The use of generative AI in pandemic prediction raises significant ethical and privacy concerns. If data is not adequately protected, the collection and processing of large amounts of personal health data can lead to potential privacy breaches. Privacy-preserving generative models based on GANs or Variational Autoencoders (VAEs) can provide privacy assurances during the data generation process [78].

Additionally, the deployment of AI models in public health decision-making must be conducted ethically, ensuring that the benefits outweigh the risks and that vulnerable populations are not disproportionately affected. The study [90] states that Generative AI offers tremendous potential in various domains but also raises critical ethical concerns. Key issues include the potential for misuse in spreading misinformation, the perpetuation of biases present in training data, the implications for privacy and data rights. It is crucial for developers, regulators and the public to collaborate in establishing robust ethical frameworks.

Table 2 List of Countries and Their Corresponding Resources

Country	Information source
Wales	https://coronavirus.data.gov.uk
Indonesia	https://covid19.go.id/peta-sebaran
Scotland	https://www.gov.scot/publications/coronavirus-covid-19-data-for-scotland
Netherlands	https://ourworldindata.org/coronavirus#explore-the-global-situation
England	https://www.england.nhs.uk/statistics/statistical-work-areas/covid-19-vaccinations
Panama	https://rainforestfoundation.org/covid-panama-gis-map

The study [91] suggests the following two solutions to address the problem of privacy leakage in generative AI models:

1. Adding a regularization term in a loss function to avoid overfitting and improve robustness; for example, this method can be applied to defend against membership inference attacks [92].
2. adding acceptable noise into the model parameters to hinder privacy inference attacks. Such methods have been used for privacy protection, particularly the combination of differential privacy and neural networks [93].

6 Conclusion

In this chapter, we observed that the integration of generative artificial intelligence in epidemic forecasting demonstrates significant progress in our ability to predict and manage disease outbreaks. Throughout this chapter, we examined how generative AI can enhance traditional epidemiological models such as SIR and SEIR, providing more accurate and timely predictions through advanced data synthesis, real-time adaptability, and comprehensive scenario simulation. The shift from conventional methods to AI-based approaches addresses many limitations such as data fragmentation, model scalability, and assumptions used in traditional approaches.

The capabilities of generative AI in integrating high-quality data, learning complex patterns, and continuously updating predictions based on new information offer significant benefits for public health. These models enable more informed decision-making that is closer to real-world conditions. Additionally, the ability to simulate various scenarios (from best-case to worst-case scenarios) provides valuable insights into potential outcomes and helps policymakers and health officials in each country prepare to address and mitigate the effects of pandemics. However, integrating generative AI into epidemic forecasting is not without challenges and limitations. Issues related to data quality, model interpretability, and ethical considerations must be carefully addressed by researchers. Ensuring the accuracy and reliability of AI predictions, increasing model transparency for easier understanding, and protecting data privacy are critical steps to building trust and ensuring the effective use of these technologies.

The continuous evolution of AI models promises further advancements in predicting and managing pandemics. Collaborative efforts between researchers and public health officials to fully leverage the potential of integrating generative AI with the medical field will be essential. By addressing current limitations and fostering innovation, we can develop stronger and more resilient systems to combat future pandemics. Generative AI's ability to integrate vast amounts of data, adapt to changing conditions, and provide accurate and actionable insights close to real-world scenarios makes it a valuable asset in public health. By embracing the potential of generative AI in the medical field, we can enhance our preparedness and response capabilities, ultimately saving lives and reducing the social impact of pandemics.

References

1. Piret J, Boivin G. Pandemics throughout history. Front Microbiol. 2021;11:631736.
2. Huremović D. Psychiatry of pandemics: a mental health response to infection outbreak. Springer; 2019.
3. Ng DTK, Leung JKL, Su J, Ng RCW, Chu SKW. Teachers' AI digital competencies and twenty-first century skills in the post-pandemic world. Educ Technol Res Dev. 2023;71(1):137–61.
4. Wolfe ND, Dunavan CP, Diamond J. Origins of major human infectious diseases. Nature. 2007;447(7142):279–83.
5. Grennan D. What is a pandemic? JAMA. 2019;321(9):910.
6. Morens DM, Folkers GK, Fauci AS. What is a pandemic? J Infect Dis. 2009;200(7):1018–21.
7. Enserink M. Swine flu: WHO 'really very close' to using the P word. 9 June 2009. Available at: http://blogs.sciencemag.org/science insider/2009/06/here-comes-phas.html. Accessed, vol. 24, 2009.
8. Kappler S, Wiesner L, Davis S. Pandemic preparedness and response. In: Ciottone's disaster medicine. Elsevier; 2024. p. 36–42.
9. WHO. Preparing for pandemics. [Online]. Available: https://www.who.int/westernpacific/activities/preparing-for-pandemics. Accessed 24 Aug 2024.
10. Aggarwal P, Mishra NK, Fatimah B, Singh P, Gupta A, Joshi SD. COVID-19 image classification using deep learning: advances, challenges and opportunities. Comput Biol Med. 2022;144:105350.
11. Liu X-X, Fong SJ, Dey N, Crespo RG, Herrera-Viedma E. A new SEAIRD pandemic prediction model with clinical and epidemiological data analysis on COVID-19 outbreak. Appl Intell. 2021;51:4162–98.
12. Raoult D, Mouffok N, Bitam I, Piarroux R, Drancourt M. Plague: history and contemporary analysis. J Infect. 2013;66(1):18–26.
13. Mordechai L, Eisenberg M, Newfield TP, Izdebski A, Kay JE, Poinar H. The Justinianic plague: an inconsequential pandemic? Proc Natl Acad Sci. 2019;116(51):25546–54.
14. Cunha CB, Cunha BA. Great plagues of the past and remaining questions. In: Paleomicrobiology: past human infections; 2008. p. 1–20.
15. Alfani G. Epidemics and pandemics: from the Justinianic plague to the Spanish flu. In: Handbook of cliometrics. Springer; 2024. p. 1931–65.
16. Dewing HB. Procopius: history of the wars. William Heinemann; 1914.
17. Bystrický P. The Justinian Plague in literary sources. In: Forum Historiae. Časopis a portál pre históriu a príbuzné spoločenské vedy. Historický ústav SAV; 2023. p. 11–31.
18. Jedwab R, Johnson ND, Koyama M. The economic impact of the black death. J Econ Lit. 2022;60(1):132–78.
19. Benedictow OJ. The black death, 1346–1353: the complete history. Boydell & Brewer; 2004.
20. Bramanti B, Stenseth NC, Walløe L, Lei X. Plague: a disease which changed the path of human civilization. Yersinia pestis: retrospective and perspective. Springer, Dordrecht. 2016:1–26.
21. Faruque SM, Albert MJ, Mekalanos JJ. Epidemiology, genetics, and ecology of toxigenic vibrio cholerae. Microbiol Mol Biol Rev. 1998;62(4):1301–14.
22. Snowden FM. Epidemics and society: from the black death to the present. Yale University Press; 2019.
23. Victor GS, Ahmed S. The importance of culture in managing mental health response to pandemics. In: Psychiatry of pandemics: a mental health response to infection outbreak; 2019. p. 55–64.
24. Weill F-X, et al. Genomic history of the seventh pandemic of cholera in Africa. Science. 2017;358(6364):785–9.
25. Padhan R, Prabheesh KP. The economics of COVID-19 pandemic: a survey. Econ Analysis Policy. 2021;70:220–37.
26. Ciotti M, Ciccozzi M, Terrinoni A, Jiang W-C, Wang C-B, Bernardini S. The COVID-19 pandemic. Crit Rev Clin Lab Sci. 2020;57(6):365–88.

27. Pokhrel S, Chhetri R. A literature review on impact of COVID-19 pandemic on teaching and learning. High Educ Future. 2021;8(1):133–41.
28. Sintema EJ. Effect of COVID-19 on the performance of grade 12 students: implications for STEM education. EURASIA J Math, Sci Technol Educ. 2020;16(7):em1851.
29. Maliszewska M, Mattoo A, Van Der Mensbrugghe D. The potential impact of COVID-19 on GDP and trade: a preliminary assessment. World Bank policy research working paper, no. 9211. 2020.
30. Alisherovna KM, Djamshedovna KD. After COVID-19 quality of life. Spect J Innov Reforms Develop. 2024;25:103–10.
31. Kauhanen L, et al. A systematic review of the mental health changes of children and young people before and during the COVID-19 pandemic. Eur Child Adolesc Psychiatry. 2023;32(6):995–1013.
32. Babvey P, Capela F, Cappa C, Lipizzi C, Petrowski N, Ramirez-Marquez J. Using social media data for assessing children's exposure to violence during the COVID-19 pandemic. Child Abuse Negl. 2021;116:104747.
33. Banh L, Strobel G. Generative artificial intelligence. Electron Mark. 2023;33(1):63.
34. Brynjolfsson E, Li D, Raymond LR. Generative AI at work. National Bureau of Economic Research; Cambridge, MA. 2023.
35. Lehmann F, Buschek D. Examining autocompletion as a basic concept for interaction with generative AI. i-com. 2021;19(3):251–64.
36. Kalota F. A primer on generative artificial intelligence. Educ Sci. 2024;14(2):172.
37. Gupta P, Ding B, Guan C, Ding D. Generative AI: a systematic review using topic modelling techniques. Data Inform Manag. 2024;8(2):100066.
38. Goodfellow I, et al. Generative adversarial nets. Adv Neural Inf Proces Syst. 2014;27:1–6.
39. Creswell A, White T, Dumoulin V, Arulkumaran K, Sengupta B, Bharath AA. Generative adversarial networks: an overview. IEEE Signal Process Mag. 2018;35(1):53–65.
40. Goodfellow I, et al. Generative adversarial networks. Commun ACM. 2020;63(11):139–44.
41. Chakraborty T, Ujjwal Reddy KS, Naik SM, Panja M, Manvitha B. Ten years of generative adversarial nets (GANs): a survey of the state-of-the-art. Machine Learn Sci Technol. 2024;5(1):11001.
42. Wang K, Gou C, Duan Y, Lin Y, Zheng X, Wang F-Y. Generative adversarial networks: introduction and outlook. IEEE/CAA J Autom Sin. 2017;4(4):588–98.
43. Liu M-Y, Tuzel O. Coupled generative adversarial networks. Adv Neural Inf Proces Syst. 2016;29:2–5.
44. Aggarwal A, Mittal M, Battineni G. Generative adversarial network: an overview of theory and applications. Int J Inform Manag Data Insights. 2021;1(1):100004.
45. Ma S, Hu Z, Ye K, Zhang X, Wang Y, Peng H. Feasibility study of patient-specific dose verification in proton therapy utilizing positron emission tomography (PET) and generative adversarial network (GAN). Med Phys. 2020;47(10):5194–208.
46. Wang H, et al. Predicting the epidemics trend of COVID-19 using epidemiological-based generative adversarial networks. IEEE J Selected Topics Signal Process. 2022;16(2):276–88.
47. Bej A, Maulik U, Sarkar A. Time-series prediction for the epidemic trends of COVID-19 using conditional generative adversarial networks regression on country-wise case studies. SN Comput Sci. 2022;3(5):352.
48. Wang H, Ma J, Zhao Z, Jia Z, Ji Z, Wu J. Adversarial training for predicting the trend of the COVID-19 pandemic. J Database Manag (JDM). 2022;33(1):1–16.
49. Quilodrán-Casas C, Silva VLS, Arcucci R, Heaney CE, Guo Y, Pain CC. Digital twins based on bidirectional LSTM and GAN for modelling the COVID-19 pandemic. Neurocomputing. 2022;470:11–28.
50. Gupta R, Pandey G, Pal SK. Comparative analysis of epidemiological models for COVID-19 pandemic predictions. Biostat Epidemiol. 2021;5(1):69–91.
51. Zhao WX, et al. A survey of large language models. arXiv. 2023. Preprint arXiv:2303.18223.

52. Chang Y, et al. A survey on evaluation of large language models. ACM Trans Intell Syst Technol. 2024;15(3):1–45.
53. Arora A, Arora A. The promise of large language models in health care. Lancet. 2023;401(10377):641.
54. Uprety D, Zhu D, West H. ChatGPT—a promising generative AI tool and its implications for cancer care. Cancer. 2023;129(15):2284–9.
55. Vincent J. Google's AI palm 2 language model announced at I/O. The Verge. Washington, DC 2023. 2023.
56. Gilson A, et al. How does ChatGPT perform on the United States Medical Licensing Examination (USMLE)? The implications of large language models for medical education and knowledge assessment. JMIR Med Educ. 2023;9(1):e45312.
57. Clynch N, Kellett J. Medical documentation: part of the solution, or part of the problem? A narrative review of the literature on the time spent on and value of medical documentation. Int J Med Inform. 2015;84(4):221–8.
58. Harrer S. Attention is not all you need: the complicated case of ethically using large language models in healthcare and medicine. EBioMedicine. 2023;90:104512.
59. Yang R, Tan TF, Lu W, Thirunavukarasu AJ, Ting DSW, Liu N. Large language models in health care: development, applications, and challenges. Health Care Sci. 2023;2(4):255–63.
60. Shao Y, et al. Hybrid value-aware transformer architecture for joint learning from longitudinal and non-longitudinal clinical data. J Personal Med. 2023;13(7):1070.
61. Ding X, Carik B, Gunturi US, Reyna V, Rho EHR. Leveraging prompt-based large language models: predicting pandemic health decisions and outcomes through social media language. In: Proceedings of the CHI conference on human factors in computing systems. 2024. p. 1–20.
62. Liu F, et al. A medical multimodal large language model for future pandemics. NPJ Digit Med. 2023;6(1):226.
63. Agarwal K, et al. Preparing for the next pandemic via transfer learning from existing diseases with hierarchical multi-modal BERT: a study on COVID-19 outcome prediction. Sci Rep. 2022;12(1):10748.
64. Liu F, et al. A multimodal large language modelling deep learning framework for the future pandemic. NPJ Digit Med. 2023;6:226.
65. Yang HF, Du H, Zhao J, et al. Advancing real-time pandemic forecasting using large language models: a COVID-19 case study. Research Square. (Version 1), 2024. https://doi.org/10.21203/rs.3.rs-4244182/v1.
66. Yang J, et al. Automating biomedical literature review for rapid drug discovery: leveraging GPT-4 to expedite pandemic response. Int J Med Inform. 2024;189:105500. https://doi.org/10.1016/j.ijmedinf.2024.105500.
67. Joloudari JH, et al. BERT-deep CNN: state of the art for sentiment analysis of COVID-19 tweets. Soc Netw Anal Min. 2023;13(1):99. https://doi.org/10.1007/s13278-023-01102-y.
68. Reddy S. Generative AI in healthcare: an implementation science informed translational path on application, integration and governance. Implement Sci. 2024;19(1):27.
69. Hwang E, Yu S. Modeling and forecasting the COVID-19 pandemic with heterogeneous autoregression approaches: South Korea. Result Phys. 2021;29:104631.
70. Rajab K, Kamalov F, Cherukuri AK. Forecasting COVID-19: vector autoregression-based model. Arab J Sci Eng. 2022:1–10.
71. Sioofy Khoojine A, Shadabfar M, Hosseini VR, Kordestani H. Network autoregressive model for the prediction of COVID-19 considering the disease interaction in neighboring countries. Entropy. 2021;23(10):1267.
72. Melin P, Monica JC, Sanchez D, Castillo O. Retraction note: a new prediction approach of the COVID-19 virus pandemic behavior with a hybrid ensemble modular nonlinear autoregressive neural network. Springer; 2023.
73. Maassen JP. The SIR and SEIR epidemiological models revisited. USA. 2020. https://doi.org/10.20944/preprints202005.0090.v1.

74. Kermack WO, McKendrick AG. A contribution to the mathematical theory of epidemics. Proc R Soc London Series A, Containing Papers Math Phys Character. 1927;115(772):700–21.
75. Chan YT. The macroeconomic impacts of the COVID-19 pandemic: a SIR-DSGE model approach. China Econ Rev. 2022;71:101725.
76. Singh P, Gupta A. Generalized SIR (GSIR) epidemic model: an improved framework for the predictive monitoring of COVID-19 pandemic. ISA Trans. 2022;124:31–40.
77. Castillo-Chavez C, Feng Z. Mathematical models for the disease dynamics of tuberculosis. New York, USA. 1996.
78. Kamrujjaman M, Saha P, Islam MS, Ghosh U. Dynamics of SEIR model: A case study of COVID-19 in Italy. Results in Control and Optimization. USA. 2020. https://doi.org/10.20944/preprints202004.0378.v1.
79. Xu C, Yu Y, Ren G, Sun Y, Si X. Stability analysis and optimal control of a fractional-order generalized SEIR model for the COVID-19 pandemic. Appl Math Comput. 2023;457:128210.
80. Patel N, Trivedi S, Chatterjee JM. Cmbatting COVID-19: artificial intelligence technologies & challenges. ScienceOpen. 2022. Preprints.
81. Sorzano COS. The mathematics of contagious diseases and their limitations in forecasting. arXiv. 2021. Preprint arXiv:2111.05727.
82. Ferguson NM. Strategies for mitigating an influenza pandemic. Nature. 2006;103:5935–40.
83. Raghavendra Rao A, Samanta D. A real-time approach with deep learning for pandemic management. In: Healthcare informatics for fighting COVID-19 and future epidemics. Springer, Cham. 2022. p. 113–39.
84. Chen X, Chong WF, Feng R, Zhang L. Pandemic risk management: resources contingency planning and allocation. Insur Math Econ. 2021;101:359–83.
85. Laventhal N, et al. The ethics of creating a resource allocation strategy during the COVID-19 pandemic. Pediatrics. 2020;146(1).
86. Ganesan S, Subramani D. Spatio-temporal predictive modeling framework for infectious disease spread. Sci Rep. 2021;11(1):6741.
87. Li C, Yao K, Wang J, Diao B, Xu Y, Zhang Q. Interpretable generative adversarial networks. In: Proceedings of the AAAI conference on artificial intelligence, 2022, p. 1280–88.
88. Gupta S. Agency, trust, and interpretability of generative adversarial networks (GANs), 2021, PhD thesis, North Carolina State University.
89. Rotulo A, et al. Mind the gap: data availability, accessibility, transparency, and credibility during the COVID-19 pandemic, an international comparative appraisal. PLOS Glob Public Health. 2023;3(4):e0001148.
90. Zlateva P, Steshina L, Petukhov I, Velev D. A conceptual framework for solving ethical issues in generative artificial intelligence. In: Electronics, communications and networks. IOS Press; 2024. p. 110–9.
91. Chen Y, Esmaeilzadeh P. Generative AI in medical practice: in-depth exploration of privacy and security challenges. J Med Internet Res. 2024;26:e53008.
92. Nasr M, Shokri R, Houmansadr A. Machine learning with membership privacy using adversarial regularization. In: Proceedings of the 2018 ACM SIGSAC conference on computer and communications security, 2018, p. 634–46.
93. Abadir PM, et al. The promise of AI and technology to improve quality of life and care for older adults. Nature Aging. 2023;3(6):629–31.

Application of GenAI in Synthetic Data Generation in the Healthcare System

Amirfarhad Farhadi and Alireza Taheri

Abbreviations

API	Application Programming Interface
EHR	Electronic Health Record
GAN	Generative Adversarial Network
GDPR	General Data Protection Regulation
GenAI	Generative Artificial Intelligence
HIPAA	Health Insurance Portability and Accountability Act
MIA	Membership Inference Attack
ML	Machine Learning
SDG	Synthetic Data Generation
VAE	Variational Autoencoder

1 Introduction

Substantial amounts of data are required for education and research in the field of healthcare. Obtaining and processing patients' data is subject to strict privacy regulations and ethical considerations. There are certain rules and regulations when it comes to handling EHRs that all companies, organizations, and medical centers must comply with in order to safely use and store patients' data. The laws associated with medical information vary across countries with relatively different policies. The Health Insurance Portability and Accountability Act (HIPAA) in the United States and the General Data Protection Regulation (GDPR) in the European union are two examples that control and limit access for safeguarding the patient's personal information [1]. Research in this field raises important concerns when sharing and using medical data. The rise of AI solutions has intensified concerns about

A. Farhadi (✉) · A. Taheri
Department of Computer Engineering, Science and Research Branch, Islamic Azad University, Tehran, Iran
e-mail: amir.farhadi@srbiau.ac.ir; alirezataheri@srbiau.ac.ir

A. Zamanifar, M. Faezipour (eds.), *Application of Generative AI in Healthcare Systems*, https://doi.org/10.1007/978-3-031-82963-5_3

protecting sensitive information. Most machine learning methods and deep neural network models are data hungry, always requiring more data to be more accurate and perform better. There are ethical concerns that need to be addressed for these models for being implemented and used in the field of healthcare. The training data used for these models should be clean and anonymized to preserve the privacy of patients. Creators and designers of AI models also need to ensure that the models are fully compliant with regulations and do not disclose any sensitive patient information.

To address the aforementioned issue, there are certain solutions that can reduce or eliminate the risk of sensitive data disclosure. Before making the data available for use, we can mask certain parts of the information in order to prevent personal data leakage. De-identification using perturbation techniques and directly editing data has proven not effective enough in preserving privacy and can even reduce utility [2, 3]. Transformation-based methods use different approaches to anonymize the data and ensure data protection. However, transformations might degrade data quality and truthfulness, which makes it less suitable for research [1]. On the other hand, new data can be generated based on the real data available to reduce the risk of privacy violations. Generative-based methods encompass a range of techniques that can generate synthetic data that closely resembles real data and mostly preserve statistical properties.

Generative Artificial intelligence (GenAI) models are trained on massive amounts of data to be able to generate myriad data types including text, images, video, and music. Besides their ability in content generation, these models are capble of a wide range of tasks. Generative models are utilized in Internet of Things for tasks such as wireless network management [4] as well as domain adaptation to transfer knowledge between domains especially when data is scarce [5, 6]. They also enhance recommender systems [7], provide lower dimensional representations [8], and more. These models require large datasets of high-quality and quantity so that they can gain insights about the data and its underlying relationships to perform well on real-world situations. Numerous industries and organizations can leverage the outstanding capabilities of GenAI to solve various problems and facilitate workflows. The rapid advancement of GenAI has revolutionized various industries, including healthcare. The healthcare industry can employ these AI models for streamlining processes, drug discovery, documentation, resource management, diagnosis, etc. The sensitivity of the data in this field requires careful handling of Electronic Health Records (EHR) to preserve patients' identity, medical information, and privacy. Research in healthcare needs data to be shared and transferred across organizations both within and outside the countries of origin. Without proper regulations and means, sensitive information may leak and the privacy of the patients will be jeopardized. GenAI models are highly suitable for synthetic data generation as they possess outstanding abilities in understanding data such as text and images. GenAI can empower synthetic data generation by creating high-quality data while preserving the essential patterns inherent in the original dataset. These models can be employed for educational and scientific simulations without disclosing critical private data.

After obtaining the required ground truth or original data, generative models can be used to learn different characteristics of the real data and then generate the relevant information based on the trained knowledge [1]. Although GenAI models can be effectively used for Synthetic Data Generation (SDG), they may accidentally pick up and repeat certain unique features from the original data. This could lead to the discovery of private information or even the reconstruction of the original data [9]. The inherent bias in the training data is still a challenge that might be addressed by sampling techniques and solely focusing on the target class. However, sampling techniques might lose the true patterns and distributions of the real data or lead to losing valuable information. Biases in the data can also be resolved by SDG algorithms along while preserving privacy and statistical resemblance [10].

The more data available for research and education, the broader the knowledge of information systems will be. However, sharing medical data requires consent or waivers to prevent violating regulations [3]. In this regard, SDG techniques play a crucial role in providing adequate data for different academic and research purposes. The synthetic data can be published through various channels, including providing clients with an Application Programming Interface (API) that can query the GenAI models to generate new data, or publishing the model itself or the ready-to-use generated data [11]. Mostly, the synthetic data created by a generative model can be used to augment the available datasets to improve performance in downstream tasks and various applications [12]. Replacing entire real datasets with synthetic ones might not always be recommended as it can compromise trust in the healthcare system, amplify bias, or risk quality features of the data such as representativeness.

In this chapter, we will review the GenAI applications in synthetic data generation for the healthcare system. There is active research in this field that has led to significant advancements in the creation of realistic and diverse synthetic healthcare datasets. We present common generative models that are used for generating synthetic data for various applications and downstream tasks. The rest of this chapter is organized in the following sections: Sect. 2 introduces GANs and VAEs as two common and powerful neural network architectures in their basic forms. Section 3 explores the different applications of synthetic data in healthcare. Section 4 will showcase specific models, frameworks, and use cases, highlighting their effectiveness in different areas. The general challenges and considerations of generating and using synthetic data are discussed in Sect. 5. Finally, Sect. 6 concludes this chapter.

2 GANs and VAEs

There are different types of generative models that each has their own strengths and weaknesses. Generative models generally have useful features that make them usable for a wide range of tasks. GANs and VAEs are two powerful types of neural networks that are commonly used to generate high-quality synthetic data in any domain given a sufficient amount of training data. These models have stronger learning abilities, which enable them to better understand the complex patterns in real-world data. This helps to prevent problems with distribution shift, create more diverse and realistic data, and simulate the noise and uncertainty that are common in the real world data [13].

GANs [14], proposed by Goodfellow et al. can generate realistic data that can be used in many different situations [3]. The GAN architecture is shown in Fig. 1. These models encompass two neural networks that compete and collaborate with each other to perform better. The generator module generates synthetic samples and the discriminator module is responsible for distinguishing between real and generated samples. The target here is both maximizing the classification accuracy of the discriminator and minimizing the generator's loss. Promising results of this model led to it being used in numerous other studies and adapted to specific tasks. MedGAN, introduced by [2], was one of the first approaches that used GAN to learn the distribution of discrete variables such as medication, diagnoses, and medication codes. They used a GAN and an autoencoder to capture and learn the patterns in real EHR data. Despite GAN's benefits and capabilities in generating content, there are several disadvantages to using them. Most notably, vanishing gradient problem happens when the gradients that are used to update the weights of the network become extremely small to a degree that it hinders the learning process and limits the development of the generator. Mode collapse, another major challenge in training GANs, happens when the generated data lose diversity and fail to represent real-world data. Several approaches and methods have been introduced to mitigate these problems in various studies.

VAEs [15] were introduced in 2013 and are capable of learning and replicating the underlying data distribution. They work by learning a lower-dimensional representation of the input that contains the essential features of the data, and then use this latent representation to reconstruct the original sample. As illustrated in Fig. 2, VAEs employ an encoder module to convert the input to a latent space (bottleneck),

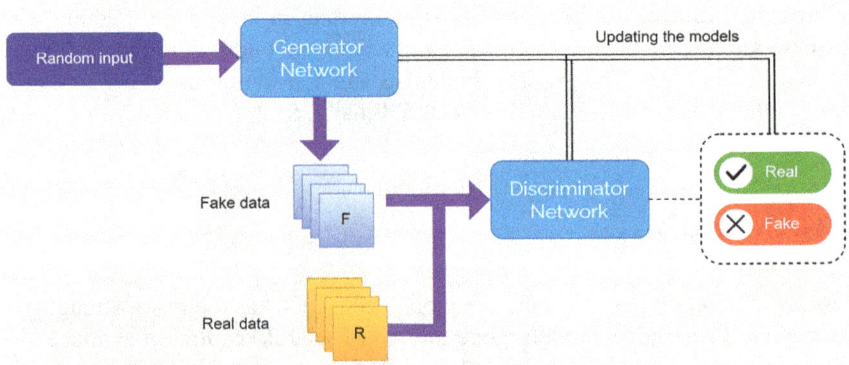

Fig. 1 GAN architecture overview

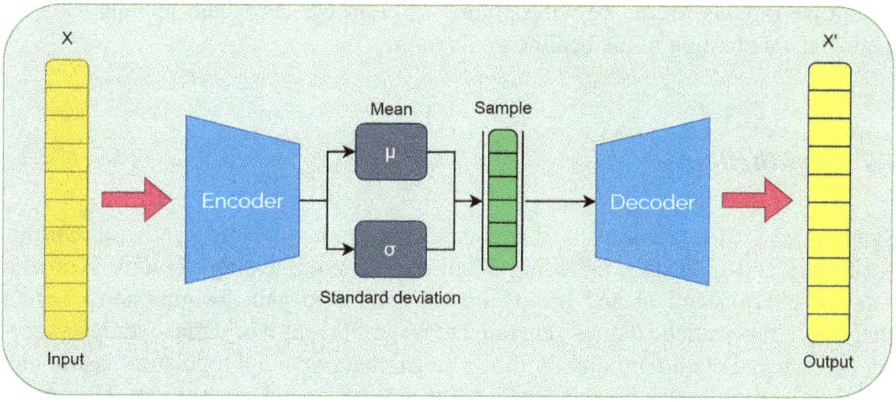

Fig. 2 The core components of a VAE

and a decoder module to transform the latent representation into the output, which resembles the input. These models are effective in representation learning and can synthesize samples by capturing the distribution of the data [16]. They can be utilized for a wide range of data types including images, audio, and text. Although VAEs are capable of learning a compressed version of the data, they tend to produce noisy low quality output [17]. Being relatively more complex than GANs, they require more data for training and better convergence.

3 Use Cases

Various models and methods have been developed to target different tasks and areas of medical synthetic data generation. The healthcare domain demands strict standards for data quality and patient privacy, as the accuracy and reliability of synthetic data directly impact patient care and outcomes in downstream tasks such as diagnosis, treatment planning, and drug discovery. There are libraries and platforms to gather different models and allow researchers and clinicians to easily access synthetic data by reducing the burden of training and fine-tuning processes and accessing proper data. Medigan [18] is an open-source Python library that enables restricted data sharing within the community along with the investigation of generative model evaluation metrics. However, to expand the available choices of generative models, researchers and clinicians still should manually explore and find the appropriate generative model best suited for their tasks as these libraries might be only focused on certain architectures. For instance, Medigan is only focused on GAN based generative models, with the promise of adding other types of models in the future. These libraries aim to save a considerable amount of time and effort spent on training generative networks and also reduce the carbon footprint of these generative models. Here, we will explore different use cases and models for synthetic data generation in the healthcare domain.

3.1 Syntheticus

Syntheticus [19] is a company that focuses on producing safe synthetic data for businesses and industries including healthcare. It provides high-quality synthetic data for pharmaceutical and healthcare companies to gain insights and conduct analysis. This synthetic data is generated to resemble real-world data while preserving privacy and confidentiality. It allows researchers to avoid regulatory issues and security risks while still having access to the data they need for research. The generated data can be employed for improving AI models performance, facilitate sharing, and enable exploration, thereby reducing costs and risks of data breaches. Syntheticus provides a fast way of accessing real-world simulated data for easing data gathering processes in research. Legal compliance is an important consideration for Syntheticus, ensuring adherence to relevant regulations and ethical standards.

3.2 Databricks

Databricks facilitates the generation of synthetic patient data using GANs, which helps address data scarcity, protect patient privacy, and enable scenario simulations without compromising real patient data. This platform combines different kinds of healthcare data, like medical records, images, and genetic information, into one place. Databricks offers a robust platform for processing and analyzing healthcare data, providing scalability, collaboration, and strong security features [20]. By leveraging Databricks, healthcare organizations can fully harness their data to enhance patient outcomes through insightful analysis, innovation, and improved results.

Databricks offers a comprehensive platform for the innovative use of synthetic data to foster collaboration, protect privacy, and enhance research capabilities. It allows efficient handling of large volumes of medical data using a distributed computing framework, enabling rapid data processing across multiple nodes. It also fosters collaboration between health researchers and data scientists through shared notebooks and version control, enhancing teamwork across disciplines. Databricks support various data types on a single platform and prioritizes data security and compliance with HIPAA and GDPR. The reliability of synthetic data is validated through statistical analysis, feature comparison, benchmarking against real data, and expert evaluation, ensuring its applicability in healthcare research.

3.3 GenRocket

GenRocket is a data generation platform with excellent capabilities in providing synthesized data with the help of GenAi for various stages of projects such as training, testing, and compliance. GenRocket empowers various industries to drive innovation while safeguarding sensitive information. In the healthcare sector, organizations can generate synthetic patient data to fuel research and development, all while adhering to stringent data privacy regulations. By rapidly producing high-quality, secure synthetic data, GenRocket enables the healthcare system to enhance the quality of services without compromising data integrity or security. This platform gives the users the opportunity to synthesize realistic data based on their preferences by controlling the volume and output format. It also focuses on enhancing the test phase by automatically providing high-quality test data that can improve the efficiency and accuracy of testing processes.

3.4 GANerAID

Clinical trials, crucial for developing new medicines and treatments, often struggle to recruit enough participants. Real patient data, while valuable, comes with privacy risks and is difficult to share. GANerAid [21] uses artificial intelligence to create realistic, but fictional, patient data for use in clinical trials. Learning from Real Data, GANerAid is trained on a dataset of real patient information, learning the patterns and characteristics of that data. Once trained, GANerAid can create new, artificial patient records that closely resemble the real data, but without containing any actual personal information. GANerAID generates data that doesn't contain any personally identifiable information, eliminating the risk of exposing sensitive patient data. Researchers can share this synthetic data more easily, enabling faster collaboration and research progress. Additionally, GANerAid can generate vast amounts of data, overcoming the limitations of small or hard-to-reach patient populations. Researchers can use GANerAid to create data representing a variety of patient profiles, including those with rare conditions or from underrepresented groups, leading to more inclusive clinical trials. In essence, GANerAid offers a powerful tool for accelerating medical research while upholding patient privacy and ethical considerations.

3.5 EHR-M-GAN

Li et al. [22] developed a novel generative AI model specifically designed to create synthetic, yet realistic, longitudinal EHRs. The model effectively handles the diverse and interconnected nature of EHR data, including demographics, diagnoses, medications, and lab results. It captures the temporal aspect of patient journeys, generating data that reflects how health conditions and treatments change over time. This study highlights a promising approach to overcome data limitations in healthcare AI by leveraging advanced generative models to create realistic and privacy-preserving synthetic EHRs.

3.6 SynTEG

EHR records are usually sequential and contain both visits and events. Zhang et al. [3] presented Synthetic Temporal EHR Generator (SynTEG) that aims to create time-based records of diagnosis. They first identified temporal patterns in clinical events, and then used GANs to generate synthetic EHRs based on the extracted patterns. SynTEG generates samples that represent temporal characteristics and features of the original data. To evaluate the usefulness of the generated data in forecasting future events, they trained two models on real and synthetic data. The similar prediction performance demonstrated the ability of the generated data to represent the real EHRs. The extent of attackers' ability to gain insights about patients' data that might be revealed by SynTEG (features and existence of certain records referred to as membership) is low and negligible. Therefore, the privacy of the sensitive patients medical records is preserved.

3.7 SynthEye

Rare eye diseases are very challenging to diagnose since data scarcity has inhibited experts from fully understanding these diseases. Veturi et al. [23] targeted Inherited Retinal Diseases (IRD), which includes a wide range of visual impairments. The accuracy of deep learning models, which assist doctors in diagnosing this disease is limited because of the natural class imbalance in training datasets. Data augmentation using various image transformations has moderate effect of model performance. They used StyleGAN2 by NVIDIA for creating Fundus Autofluorescence (FAF) images that are used to help with genetic diagnosis. The Moorfields Eye Hospital IRD dataset with 1800 patients FAF images is utilized in this study for evaluation. Three metrics were investigated to assess the quality of the generated images. They evaluated visual and distribution similarity in addition to generalizability meaning that the images should not be merely copies of the training dataset. The results suggested that SynthEye was able to generate images of high-quality, which are similar but not copies of real data. Although, this generative model could not improve the classification performance of downstream tasks, the models trained on only synthetic data showed similar classification performance. This shows that the generated data closely resembles the patterns and the distribution of the original dataset.

3.8 ScoEHR

Naseer et al. [24] aimed to solve the EHR accessibility issues, including expenses, ethical and regulatory concerns, and time constraints. There are many machine learning applications such as diagnosis and detection that can benefit from diverse synthetic EHRs. ScoEHR uses a combination of an autoencoder with a diffusion model to produce high-quality images with good mode coverage. This method achieved better results regarding the quality of the synthetic data compared to other baselines on two datasets. Different evaluation metrics such as Log-cluster, dimensional distribution, pairwise correlation difference, and synthetic ranking agreement were used to assess and compare different SDG methods. Moreover, they used clinician evaluation in which they provided three expert clinicians with 100 records of both real and synthetic data and a set of instructions for labeling them. The clinicians were asked to label each patient medical records as realistic or unrealistic. The results show that ScoEHR achieves the best performance compared with SOTA methods. Additionally, the generated data showed little risk of privacy violation and membership inference attack (MIA).

3.9 MedGen3D

Medical image generation is usually conducted in two dimensions for various applications. 3D images on the other hand, are useful in segmentation and detection [25]. Generating 3D images has different challenges including GPU memory constraints that can be addressed by lowering the quality and resolution. MedGen3D [26] views data as sequences of slices and uses a multi-step procedure for creating realistic 3D medical images. In this approach, a mask is first generated using a specialized model that leverages a combination of conditional and unconditional generation processes. The mask acts as a blueprint that will be used to create the final image. The image generator in this study is conditioned on the generated masks that can create realistic images with respect to the masks that preserves the spatial relationship consistent between consecutive slices of data. This model has proved helpful in generating image-mask pairs with limited annotated data.

3.10 EHR-Safe

EHR data are heterogeneous, containing numerical and categorical features. These records can be highly non-uniform with varying distributions and characteristics. To address this issue, Yoon et al. [27] have proposed EHR-safe to preserve the privacy of patients while resembling real-data patterns. They employed an encoder-decoder architecture that helps a GAN to model heterogeneous EHR data. One-hot encoding of categorical features might be solution to handle this type of data. However, for features like medical codes that can have a large number of unique values, one-hot encoding will lead to high dimensional representations, which will reduce efficiency. For mitigating this issue, the categorical data is first one-hot encoded and then transformed into a latent space. Moreover, to address the problem of mode collapse, which happens when GANs fail to generalize the generated features and diversify, they used a stochastic normalization for numerical values. Using this approach the numerical values that can be of non-uniform distributions will be mapped to a new distribution with respect to ratios of unique values, which will eventually make it easier for GANs to model. The statistical similarity and utility of the generated samples of EHR-Safe are almost the same as the original data while preserving the patient's privacy.

3.11 MTGAN

Each patient can have multiple visits in real-world clinical records. Diagnoses during each visit are mostly correlated over time. GANs can produce independent visit data that can then be attached together to form a sequence. However, this method cannot preserve temporal correlation between visits. Lu et al. [28] proposed a Multi-label Time-series GAN (MTGAN) to address the aforementioned issue and also consider rare diseases in the generated data. This method aims to create realistic samples of medical records that preserve the connections between the visits. Using Gated Recurrent Units (GRUs), they generated diagnosis probabilities by a next visit prediction approach. To make sure that uncommon diseases have the chance to be generated in visit sequences, they used a smooth conditional matrix. Unlike using a conditional vector that can be concatenated directly with the noise vector of the generator, they considered using a matrix to avoid extreme cases of the rare diseases occurring in the first or all the visits. The experimental results show that MTGAN is able to generate high-quality synthetic data with enhanced statistical properties that can improve performance of downstream prediction tasks.

3.12 CorGAN

Torfi et al. [29] proposed Correlation-capturing Generative Adversarial Network (CorGAN) that captures the correlations between features for generating realistic synthetic medical records. They used minibatch discrimination to mitigate mode collapse, common issue in GANs. For handling discrete values, CorGAN utilizes a pre-trained convolutional autoencoder (CAE). The CAE is trained to convert discrete values into a latent representation, and then transform them back to discrete values. The decoder part of this CAE is leveraged to convert the generator's continuous values into discrete values. To ensure that the discriminator receives discrete values, the output values of the decoder are rounded to the nearest integer. The membership inference attack is considered to assess the privacy implications of the generated data. This type of attack refers to the ability of an adversary in determining whether a particular individual's data was used in the training process. As demonstrated by the results, CorGAN was able to generate similar synthetic data while preserving patients from identification. It also proved that using Convolutional Neural Networks (CNN) for capturing the correlations is more effective than Multilayer Perceptrons (MLP).

3.13 Bt-GAN

Fairness is a concept related to bias that when used for synthetic data means that any model trained on the generated data can make fair predictions in real-world scenarios. Bias-transforming Generative Adversarial Network (Bt-GAN) by Ramachandranpillai et al. [30] is a framework that addresses fairness in downstream tasks and controls bias amplification in SDG. There are multiple techniques employed to capture the right data distribution and avoid correlation biases. To handle missing values and partially labeled records, a special type of GAN named Triple GAN, with an additional classifier is utilized. The bias-transform stage is conducted by fine-tunning the generator using a fairness penalty to a generate fair distribution. The experimental results demonstrate that this method generates data with minimum bias compared to other baselines. Bt-GAN can successfully balance fairness and utility with high precision and recall.

3.14 DP-ACTGAN

Luo [9] proposed framework named Differentially Private Auxiliary Classifier Conditional Tabular Generative Adversarial Network (DP-ACTGAN) for generating high-quality synthetic data and mitigating privacy breaches in its architecture. Differential privacy is utilized by adding Gaussian noise to the to the discriminator gradient to prevent the generated data from being used to identify or learn information about individuals. A classifier with a fully connected network is used to evaluate the generated samples and ensure that they resemble the real data. This classifier is trained on real data and its labels, enabling it to help the generator to create samples that are more similar to the original data. DOMIAS [31] is used in this study as a tool for investigating privacy risks in the generated data. This model helps designers of generative models gain valuable insights into challenges that might endanger patient safety and privacy. DP-ACTGAN can generate synthetic data that follows the statistical patterns of the real samples while protecting individuals' privacy in data sharing and utilization.

3.15 CTGAN

Xu et al. [32] proposed a Conditional Tabular Generative Adversarial Network (CTGAN), which is focused on generating tabular data. This model employs a technique called mode-specific normalization for converting continuous features with various ranges into a constrained vector space. This technique eliminates the complicated distributions, which makes the data easier for the generator to model. Moreover, random sampling might hinder the proper representation of minority categories. The generator module of the GAN is designed to be conditional, taking a conditional vector as input. The conditional GAN can be used to address the class imbalance problem. CTGAN can be used to generate synthetic tabular data by learning the properties of columns with random distributions. Bietsch et al. [33] used CTGAN for improving the patient's length of stay (LOS). Hospitals and insurance companies can benefit by predicting the inpatient LOS as they can enhance the quality of their service and efficiently manage resources. They categorized numerical values showing the days a patient stayed in the hospital to short, medium, and long categories. They then used the synthesized tabular EHR to train and evaluate three ML models, Support Vector Machine (SVM), K-Nearest Neighbor, and Random Forest. CTGAN showed decent capability in generating data with the same distribution for different columns. However, this study found that using synthetic data generated by this model for LOS detection is challenging and requires more improvement especially for highly imbalanced real data with missing values.

3.16 DP-CGANS

Early access to data in research is critical to know whether the data is actually useful for answering research question. If the data is relevant for the project, researchers can start requesting access to the data and comply with legal requirements. To tackle this problem and create synthetic data that is statistically and structurally similar to the real data, Sun et al. [34] have proposed Differentially Private-Conditional Generative Adversarial Networks (DP-CGANS). This model starts by separating the real data into two categories of: continuous and categorical, for better generator performance. Categorical variables are one-hot encoded and continuous variables are normalized before being fed to the generator. To prevent the loss of the information and dependencies between variables, they condition the generator with a vector to represent the dependencies and relationships between different variables. This approach leverages differential privacy to preserve the privacy of individuals in the real dataset. Differential privacy is implemented by adding noise using a Gaussian additive noise mechanism. A GAN model is used for generation phase and the Gaussian noise is used for training the discriminator, which will eventually affect the generator as well. After generating differentially private synthetic data, the transformation on the variables is reversed to restore the original representation of the data. In terms of downstream tasks performance, statistical resemblance, and privacy protection, DP-CGANS achieved superior performance compared to baseline generative models.

3.17 *KDE-KNN*

Macias-Fassio et al. [35] have proposed a novel approach for synthetic data generation named Kernel Density Estimator and K-Nearest Neighbors sampling (KDE-KNN). They aim to improve early disease diagnosis and focus specifically on sepsis. Sepsis is a condition in which the body fails to respond properly to an infection. Predicting this condition is critical and challenging as it progresses rapidly and can become dangerous. They used multivariate KDE to approximate the probability density function of the original dataset features along with the dependencies and relationships between them. KDE is trained on two categories of data, which are patients with or without sepsis. Then sampling process creates synthetic data by selecting from the generated probability distribution. Now a KNN model that is trained on the provided dataset is used to validate the synthetic data. They used mean Distance to Closest Record (DCR) metric to investigate the privacy protection level of the generated data, which works by calculating the distance between synthetic and real samples. Downstream sepsis detection models achieved better performance using KDE-KNN generated balanced datasets than original real samples. The balanced number of patients with or without sepsis in the datasets is deemed to be the major contributing factor to have more accurate models.

4 Applications

Synthetic data is artificially created information, distinct from data collected through real-world events and direct observation. Data professionals employ algorithms to produce synthetic data from existing datasets, carefully setting parameters to ensure it meets the necessary quality standards for its intended applications. This type of data can either supplement existing datasets that are insufficient on their own or replace real-world datasets that are difficult to access or use, such as those subject to strict regulations. Synthetic data can also fill gaps where real-world data is unavailable, such as in analyzing rare, theoretical, or futuristic scenarios that lack empirical data. Additionally, analysts can use synthetic data to simulate real-world situations that are too risky or hazardous to replicate directly.

GenAI models have emerged as powerful tools for SDG. There are various challenges that can be addressed using synthetic data. Many tasks can also be facilitated by utilizing high-quality generated data. The first major responsibility of the generated data is always privacy preservation and identity protection. This makes health related tasks that use sensitive medical information fully comply with strict regulations regarding handling EHRs. Preventing patients' identity form being compromised by malicious intents, is the top priority. Therefore, we can consider privacy protection as a basic requirement for any synthetic data generation process in healthcare, and dedicate this section to other applications that can benefit from the use of synthetic data.

4.1 Data Augmentation

One of the well-known applications of synthetic data is using it to boost the performance of machine learning models or even as extra data for research. In order to increase the generalizability and accuracy of ML models for different tasks, additional data can be used to diversify and extend the original dataset [36]. Data augmentation has long been used in the field as a solution to data scarcity that limits the accuracy of research [37]. Clinical trial costs and certain regulations associated with patient's data, led Zhu et al. [38] to propose a framework for generating glucose time series data. Obtaining large-scale personalized data requires adherence to regulations and preserving privacy of the patients, which usually comes with high costs and is time-consuming. GlueGAN can generate high-quality synthetic personalized data for augmenting the available datasets. Moreover, structured EHR consists of various data types and formats. The recorded medical data can be in forms of time-series or tabular that each can contain several data types such as discrete, categorical and continuous. According to the requirements, any combination of these formats and types can be used together in EHRs. Additionally, depending on the patient's treatment and medical services provided to them, different sections of healthcare services might appear in their medical records. GenAI can help produce synthetic EHR that preserve identity and privacy while resembling real-world patient records for myriad applications [17]. As medical records contain various types of data in different forms, generative models should be able to synthesize data with high fidelity that maintains the characteristics, distributions, and consistency of the original data, to make the generated data suitable for augmenting original datasets. Adversarial networks especially GANs are also widely used for data augmentation by generating realistic data [39].

4.2 Bias Correction

Besides data augmentation that can be vital in many scenarios, constructing a less biased dataset can be one of the useful applications of SDG. Biased datasets are unbalanced and represent certain groups or classes unfairly, which will make decisions in downstream tasks less accurate. For example, in a dataset where diabetes disease samples are mostly for Asian ethnicity, the effect of neglecting other ethnicity groups might adversely affect the results of any research on that data. Making secondary datasets out of the unbalanced ones through sampling is an effective solution that has been used by researchers for a long time. Downsampling the majority class or adding more data for the underrepresented group can correct the bias in the data. Nonetheless, valuable information will be lost during downsampling, which will lead to performance reduction [40]. This bias can easily appear in any dataset due to a lack of representation or problems in sampling. In the domain of healthcare this bias can occur for features like gender, disease, race, ethnicity, location, or any other characteristic of the data. GenAI can effectively mitigate this bias by reading and understanding the patterns and relationship among the data and generate new samples that mimics the real data. This way researchers can have access to more data that is partially synthetic but is well balanced and fairly represent the diverse population of patients. However, certain risks in bias mitigation should be concerned when adding new fake samples in order to preserve the original characteristics of the data and its utility. Bias amplification on the other hand can be one of the challenges that should be addressed carefully. When adding synthetic data to an existing dataset, it is critical to ensure that new samples do not introduce or amplify bias.

4.3 Data Completion

Machine learning methods' abilities in prediction and diagnosis can be hindered by the lack of EHR quality. Medical records are sometimes incomplete and contain errors and inconsistencies [41]. Missing data is one of the major challenges of working with EHRs that can limit the AI models performance. The causes of this missingness can be different such as machine failure or inability to records data for safety reasons or high costs. Deletion might seem like a quick and effective solution for such samples. However, by removing samples that are partially useful we might lose valuable information. This can be more severe in datasets that contain large numbers of incomplete samples. In addition to generating complete samples, GenAI models are capable of completing a sample based on the records themselves and the real dataset. Data imputation using GenAI can be an effective solution for handling missing data by preserving the available information and accurate completion.

4.4 Education

By lowering the costs and risks of data provision, education and research can significantly benefit from using synthetic data. SDG offers more availability of data for researchers and students who may be limited by access to real-world datasets. GenAI can produce data for learning purposes that can be utilized in schools or research centers. The augmented data here can be used to cover specific areas that there is a lack of quality samples or where students need help [42]. For example, imagine a student who is having trouble distinguishing benign and malignant tumors. GenAI can help them by generating images of both types in different levels of severity. By training a generative model on a large number of tumor images the model can understand the relationship between the appearance of the tumor and its type. Additionally, GenAI can enhance education by enabling institutions and medical centers to share data and collaborate on different projects using de-identified safe data that is available easier.

4.5 Prototyping and Evaluation

In the case of developing medical devices, functionality evaluation, or assessing models before deployment, large scale datasets are required to confirm the performance or shift the project to the next phase. In these situations, synthetic data can be very helpful by providing faster and easier access to data. Moreover, when the required de-identified data is available but acquiring it requires large financial resources and compliance conditions, accessing ready to use data can significantly expedite project completion. Using synthetic data in these cases will speed up the process of research and development of projects, reduce costs, save time, and solve regulatory compliance issues [43].

5 Challenges and Considerations

Undoubtedly, GenAI has deeply influenced medical research and education by improving data accessibility, reducing costs, saving time, and preserving the identity and privacy of patients in the process. However, there are certain challenges and risks that might hinder its widespread adoption and effective implementation. These issues need to be addressed in order to make the most of these models while minimizing the adverse effects of their drawbacks. For example, as critical as it is for data to contain the least amount of sensitive identifiable information possible, it is important for the output data to still be useful and representative of the real-world data [10]. Other than specific issues that generative models with different designs might face, such as mode collapse, convergence problems, computational expense, and resource requirements [44], there are general aspects of the output of GenAI that must be considered before being applied and used in the field [45]. Figure 3 provides a visual representation of the critical factors and obstacles related to SDG in healthcare.

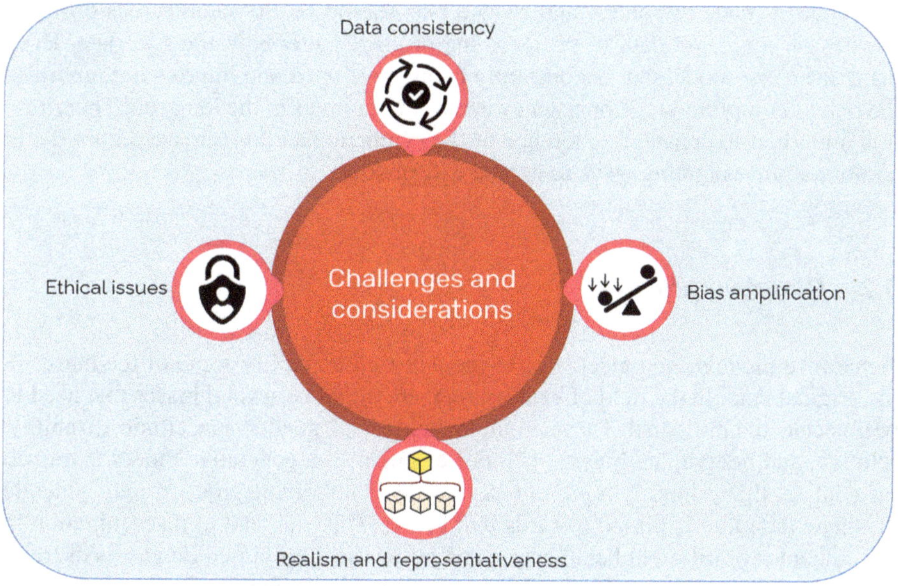

Fig. 3 Key considerations and challenges of SDG in healthcare

5.1 Data Consistency

There are various quality assessment metrics that researchers and developers of generative models exploit to evaluate synthetic data. Regardless of the thresholds and standards in place to control the generation process, it is important to maintain a logical balance and score, and keep uniform quality across the datasets [46]. For example, consider a research center that uses samples of real data which are inadequate to perform experiments or progress projects. This center can employ a generative model to fabricate data that closely resembles their original samples. They can consider a certain proportion ratio of synthetic to original data to augment their own dataset. Researchers need to carefully evaluate the augmented dataset for determining its quality. However, it should be noted that only considering a few metrics for evaluation might lead to data inconsistency. Researchers need to ensure that the new data not only achieves high scores in different metrics regarding its usability, bias, fairness, and privacy preservation, but also follows certain patterns of the real data or the older generation of samples. Consistency needs to be preserved over time to make sure that the synthetic data does not gradually deviate from the original source. This can mislead the research and create additional problems.

In cases where multiple GenAI models are used to produce enough data, there needs to be a unified standard across those models to evaluate the results. This is more prominent especially when the models are developed by different companies that may not share their evaluation metrics or even use different ones. The lack of a unified definition of synthetic data itself can further complicate the situation [37].

Every effort made to control and reduce bias should be the same across different batches of generated data to preserve the original patterns in the real data. Even using the same model that is constantly being developed and improved might raise the risk of compromising consistency across the samples in the long run. Therefore, it is important to consider coherence of the synthetic data to increase reliability, in addition to investigating ways to enhance its quality.

5.2 *Bias Amplification*

Generative models can preserve or in the worst case amplify some of the biases in the original data. In the field of healthcare, there might be several biases that need to be detected and mitigated. These might include racial, gender, age, ethnic, disability, religion, and geographic biases [47]. For example, if a generative model is trained on a dataset that primarily represents a specific demographic group, it may generate synthetic data that is biased towards that group. This can lead to discrimination in the outcomes of different healthcare applications, such as biased diagnosis or treatment recommendations [48]. While the synthetic data should resemble real-world original data, it should not amplify the bias in the training data. The inherent bias in the training dataset can be amplified in the SDG process if the model does not accurately represent the distribution of data subgroups. This can lead to the generation of synthetic data that perpetuates or exacerbates existing inequalities [45].

The black-box nature of the generative models can also contribute to introducing bias in different stages of the algorithm development process [48]. Due to the complexity and lack of transparency of these models, it can be difficult to identify and address biases that might be present in the training data or the model architecture and design. Therefore, employing techniques to gain insight into the process of decision making of these models can help improve interpretability, which will eventually increase trust in these systems too. It is imperative to control bias in every stage of the development and deployment of AI systems. Because not only do downstream tasks struggle with bias in the synthetic data, but also there are risks of reinforcing existing biases or creating new ones in designing new models. According to Abràmoff et al. [47], biases can emerge from different sources in various stages of the AI system lifecycle, which includes conception, design, development, validation, access and marketing, and monitoring. Hence, controlling bias only in synthetic data generation is not adequate and it is of vital importance to employ a comprehensive and systematic approach to bias mitigation throughout the entire AI lifecycle.

Perpetuating bias by GenAI is possible when biases in the original dataset are magnified by the model when generating data [12, 37]. For example, if the real medical records that are used to train the generative model mostly contain records of male individuals, the resultant synthetic data will mostly follow this trend, which might lead to bias amplification. The sensitivity of the patterns in health-related data requires strict analysis of the original data and the generated samples to ensure that the techniques used for mitigating bias, do not negatively impact the quality and utility of the data. These methods should not create false correlations, impact the representativeness, or limit the generalizability of the synthetic data. Therefore, it is essential to monitor and evaluate both the original and synthetic data for any unintended bias using different techniques such as anomaly detection [37].

5.3 Ethical Issues

As GenAI models progress in the field of healthcare, it becomes increasingly difficult to distinguish real data from machine-generated samples. Considering ethical issues and regulations is essential for ensuring that the generative models create data that respects patients' privacy and safety. These models are entirely trained on patients' medical records to create synthetic data with similar patterns and statistical features. Therefore, it is critical that both the models and their outputs comply with certain rules and laws. Additionally, it is of vital importance to consider the ethical implications of using synthetic data generated from patient records. If there are concerns regarding the potential misuse of synthetic data, they should be addressed before deploying these models and publishing the generated data.

The excessive use of artificial data produced by generative models might negatively influence the patients' trust in the medical system. Healthcare professionals and patients may doubt the accuracy of a model's diagnosis if it is trained mostly on synthetic, non-real data [13]. The level of transparency and interpretability can also raise trust in how GenAI models produce samples. This can be achieved by establishing standards and clear definitions that set the required level of explainability and its trade-off with performance. Additionally, providing clear documentation of the data generation process and a thorough analysis of the output might help detect potential limitations and errors in the data [37]. Moreover, while SDG is an effective way to anonymize data and preserve privacy, the generated data should not be so similar to the original data that it becomes reidentifiable. As depicted in Fig. 4, membership and attribute disclosure attacks pose significant risks to data privacy. It is important to keep a balance between ethical issues and realism [45]. When a fabricated sample closely resembles a real record of an individual, an attacker can use the synthetic data to learn or find out more about that person. Hence, it is crucial to evaluate the reidentification potential of the synthetic data before publishing it [49]. MIAs are another privacy threat that can arise in generative models, especially when trained on large datasets. In a MIA, an attacker attempts to determine whether a specific individual's data was used for training the generative model [50]. This can reveal sensitive information about patients and have serious privacy implications.

Furthermore, considering a chain of custody database for increasing integrity and security of the generated data that is about to be shared between organizations is recommended [37]. This will ensure that the data flow is controlled and potential violations can be traced throughout the entire data lifecycle. To enhance the trust and reliability of the generated data, blockchain technology and a digital chain of

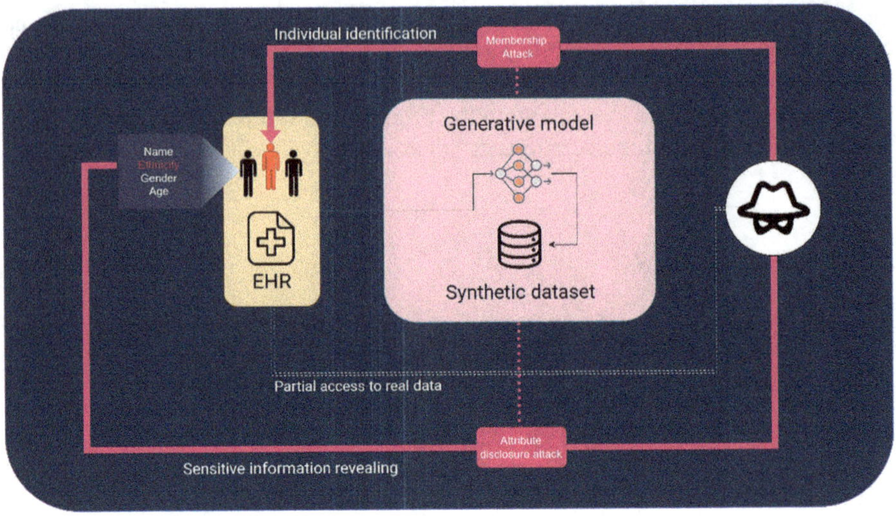

Fig. 4 Membership and attribute disclosure attacks

custody can be utilized, which allows for greater reliability, transparency, and the identification of unauthorized access and any malicious activities [51, 52].

5.4 *Realism and Representativeness*

GenAI models need to imitate real-world data by statistically resembling the underlying distributions and patterns found in genuine datasets. This ensures that the synthetic data generated is representative and can be used effectively for various tasks, such as training other models or conducting simulations. For these models to generate high-quality synthetic data, they should be exposed to large amounts of training data. Accessing a high number of patient records might not be straightforward as there are certain regulations and laws regarding handling sensitive patient information. Additionally, missing data that might appear in the training data for various reasons, can limit the accuracy of the generated synthetic data. Therefore, developers and researchers must employ necessary techniques to handle missing data or other factors that might contribute to data quality degradation. Any deviation in training data can lead to biased or inaccurate synthetic data, which can ultimately undermine the realism and representativeness of the generated samples.

Comprehensiveness of the generated data is achieved through training GenAI models on diverse and representative datasets that capture the full range of variability in real-world data. Generative models can face challenges in generating realistic and representative data for minority groups or regions with limited data availability, primarily due to insufficient training examples. In SDG, this can lead to discrimination and amplification of existing inequalities [11]. When it comes to generating new samples that should resemble the original data that the model was trained on, it is critical to consider the trade-off between resemblance and privacy. This means that by trying to generate data that exactly resembles the training dataset, the risk of overfitting and privacy violation exists [53].

It is also recommended to include training samples from different countries around the world to expand the diversity of the original data. While AI and its applications are mostly present in developed countries, it is crucial to gather as much data as possible which vary in different features to expand the generalizability of GenAI models and produce more diverse and representative data [48]. This is especially important if these AI tools are being exploited in other countries where little or no data originated from that area to contribute to training the models.

6 Conclusion

Protecting the privacy of patients is an essential rule in handling EHRs that contain their personal information. Different rules and laws supporting individuals' sensitive medical information hinder easy data access by researchers and students. Therefore, there is a need for anonymization techniques to deidentify the medical records in order to make them safe to be handed to different domestic or international institutions for various projects and education. These methods are critical in omitting the information that can be misused for identifying patients or knowing more about them. There are well known risks and attacks that can compromise patients' privacy including membership and attribute disclosure attacks. Synthetic data generation can go beyond privacy preservation by offering countless benefits to research and education, data augmentation for AI models, data loss management, and prediction. GenAI can produce synthetic data for machine learning models to boost their performance and generalizability. Clinicians can leverage these enhanced models for improving diagnosis and treatment, and patients can enjoy high-quality medical services. However, it is critical to consider the limitations and challenges of using GenAI for SDG, as these models are not perfect and there are still concerns regarding the quality of the generated data and ethical issues. SDG is still an evolving area and requires further in-depth research to address the potential limitations and risks associated with converting sensitive data to similar and safe fabricated data.

References

1. Murtaza H, et al. Synthetic data generation: state of the art in health care domain. Comput Sci Rev. 2023;48:100546.
2. Choi E, et al. Generating multi-label discrete patient records using generative adversarial networks. In: Machine learning for healthcare conference. PMLR; 2017.
3. Zhang Z, et al. SynTEG: a framework for temporal structured electronic health data simulation. J Am Med Inform Assoc. 2021;28(3):596–604.

4. Liu Y, et al. Deep generative model and its applications in efficient wireless network management: a tutorial and case study. IEEE Wirel Commun. 2024;31(4):199–207.
5. Farhadi A, Sharifi A. Leveraging meta-learning to improve unsupervised domain adaptation. Comput J. 2024;67(5):1838–50.
6. Farhadi A, et al. Domain adaptation in reinforcement learning: a comprehensive and systematic study. J Zhejiang Univ Sci C. 2024;25(11):1446–1465. https://doi.org/10.1631/FITEE.2300668.
7. Deldjoo Y, et al. A review of modern recommender systems using generative models (gen-recsys). In: Proceedings of the 30th ACM SIGKDD conference on Knowledge Discovery and Data Mining. 2024.
8. Farhadi A, et al. Unsupervised domain adaptation for image classification based on deep neural networks. Intelligent Multimedia Process Commun Syst (IMPCS). 2023;4(1):27–37.
9. Luo X. A method for privacy-safe synthetic health data. Acad J Sci Technol. 2024;10(1):445–50.
10. Kiran A, Kumar SS. A methodology and an empirical analysis to determine the most suitable synthetic data generator. IEEE Access. 2024;12:12209–28.
11. van Breugel B, van der Schaar M. Beyond privacy: navigating the opportunities and challenges of synthetic data. arXiv. 2023. Preprint arXiv:2304.03722.
12. Ktena I, et al. Generative models improve fairness of medical classifiers under distribution shifts. Nat Med. 2024:1–8.
13. Hao S, et al. Synthetic data in AI: challenges, applications, and ethical implications. arXiv. 2024. Preprint arXiv:2401.01629.
14. Goodfellow I, et al. Generative adversarial nets. Adv Neural Inf Proces Syst. 2014;27.
15. Kingma DP. Auto-encoding variational bayes. arXiv. 2013. Preprint arXiv:1312.6114.
16. Goyal M, Mahmoud QH. A systematic review of synthetic data generation techniques using generative AI. Electronics. 2024;13(17):3509.
17. Ghosheh GO, Li J, Zhu T. A survey of generative adversarial networks for synthesizing structured electronic health records. ACM Comput Surv. 2024;56(6):1–34.
18. Osuala R, et al. Medigan: a python library of pretrained generative models for medical image synthesis. J Med Imag. 2023;10(6):061403.
19. Leveraging synthetic data for innovative healthcare and pharma solutions. [cited 4 September 2024]; Available from: https://syntheticus.ai/synthetic-data-for-healthcare-and-pharma.
20. L'Esteve R. The Azure Data lakehouse toolkit: building and scaling data lakehouses on Azure with delta lake, Apache spark, databricks, synapse analytics, and snowflake. Springer; 2022.
21. Krenmayr L, et al. GANerAid: realistic synthetic patient data for clinical trials. Inform Med Unlocked. 2022;35:101118.
22. Li J, et al. Generating synthetic mixed-type longitudinal electronic health records for artificial intelligent applications. NPJ Digit Med. 2023;6(1):98.
23. Veturi YA, et al. SynthEye: investigating the impact of synthetic data on artificial intelligence-assisted gene diagnosis of inherited retinal disease. Ophthalmol Sci. 2023;3(2):100258.
24. Naseer AA, et al. ScoEHR: generating synthetic electronic health records using continuous-time diffusion models. In: Machine learning for healthcare conference. PMLR; 2023.
25. Hatamizadeh, A., et al. Unetr: Transformers for 3d medical image segmentation. In: Proceedings of the IEEE/CVF winter conference on applications of computer vision. 2022.
26. Han K, et al. Medgen3d: a deep generative framework for paired 3d image and mask generation. In: International conference on medical image computing and computer-assisted intervention. Springer; 2023.
27. Yoon J, et al. EHR-safe: generating high-fidelity and privacy-preserving synthetic electronic health records. NPJ Digit Med. 2023;6(1):141.
28. Lu C, et al. Multi-label clinical time-series generation via conditional GAN. IEEE Trans Knowl Data Eng. 2023.
29. Torfi A, Fox EA. CorGAN: correlation-capturing convolutional generative adversarial networks for generating synthetic healthcare records. In The thirty-third international flairs conference. 2020.

30. Ramachandranpillai R, et al. Bt-GAN: generating fair synthetic Healthdata via bias-transforming generative adversarial networks. J Artif Intell Res. 2024;79:1313–41.
31. Van Breugel B, et al. Membership inference attacks against synthetic data through overfitting detection. arXiv. 2023. Preprint arXiv:2302.12580.
32. Xu L, et al. Modeling tabular data using conditional gan. Adv Neural Inf Proces Syst. 2019;32.
33. Bietsch D, Stahlbock R, Voß S. Electronic health data in the context of patient length-of-stay prediction: using generative adversarial nets for synthetic data creation. In: 2023 congress in computer science, computer engineering, & applied computing (CSCE). IEEE; 2023.
34. Sun C, van Soest J, Dumontier M. Generating synthetic personal health data using conditional generative adversarial networks combining with differential privacy. J Biomed Inform. 2023;143:104404.
35. Macias-Fassio E, et al. Privacy-preserving statistical data generation: application to sepsis detection. arXiv. 2024. Preprint arXiv:2404.16638.
36. Taheri A, Zamanifar A, Farhadi A. Enhancing aspect-based sentiment analysis using data augmentation based on back-translation. Int J Data Sci Anal. 2024:1–26.
37. Giuffrè M, Shung DL. Harnessing the power of synthetic data in healthcare: innovation, application, and privacy. NPJ Digit Med. 2023;6(1):186.
38. Zhu T, et al. GluGAN: generating personalized glucose time series using generative adversarial networks. IEEE J Biomed Health Inform. 2023;27(10):5122–33.
39. Mahalegi HSM, et al. Generative adversarial networks for heterogeneous unsupervised domain adaptation detection. In: 2024 IEEE 28th international conference on intelligent engineering systems (INES). IEEE; 2024.
40. Ruiz-Casado JL, Molina-Cabello MA, Luque-Baena RM. Enhancing histopathological image classification performance through synthetic data generation with generative adversarial networks. Sensors. 2024;24(12):3777.
41. Bernardini M, et al. A novel missing data imputation approach based on clinical conditional generative adversarial networks applied to EHR datasets. Comput Biol Med. 2023;163:107188.
42. Synthetic data: a potential game changer for healthcare. 2023 [cited 1 September 2024]; Available from: https://mathco.com/article/synthetic-data-a-potential-gamechanger-for-healthcare/.
43. Richman A. Synthetic test data: critical for software testing. 2023 [cited 1 September 2024]; Available from: https://www.k2view.com/blog/synthetic-test-data/.
44. Jadon A, Kumar S. Leveraging generative ai models for synthetic data generation in healthcare: balancing research and privacy. In 2023 international conference on smart applications, communications and networking (SmartNets). IEEE; 2023.
45. Vallevik VB, et al. Can I trust my fake data–a comprehensive quality assessment framework for synthetic tabular data in healthcare. Int J Med Inform. 2024:105413.
46. Zamzmi G, et al. Scorecards for synthetic medical data evaluation and reporting. arXiv. 2024. Preprint arXiv:2406.11143.
47. Abràmoff MD, et al. Considerations for addressing bias in artificial intelligence for health equity. NPJ Digit Med. 2023;6(1):170.
48. Umer F, Adnan N. Generative artificial intelligence: synthetic datasets in dentistry. BDJ Open. 2024;10(1):13.
49. El Kababji S, et al. Evaluating the utility and privacy of synthetic breast cancer clinical trial data sets. JCO Clin Cancer Inform. 2023;7:e2300116.
50. Chen Y, Esmaeilzadeh P. Generative AI in medical practice: in-depth exploration of privacy and security challenges. J Med Internet Res. 2024;26:e53008.
51. Lataran PN, et al. Developing a BERT-enhanced blockchain model for HealthInsurance fraud detection. J Inform Syst Res Pract. 2024;2(3):56–61.
52. Farhadi A, et al. Leveraging blockchain and ANFIS for optimal supply chain management. arXiv. 2024. Preprint arXiv:2408.17161.
53. Bhanot K, et al. The problem of fairness in synthetic healthcare data. Entropy. 2021;23(9):1165.

Application of GenAI in Clinical Administration Support

Alireza Taheri, Amirfarhad Farhadi, and Azadeh Zamanifar

Abbreviations

ASR	Automatic Speech Recognition
BIRP	Behavior, Intervention, Response, and Plan
CPT	Current Procedural Terminology
EHR	Electronic Health Record
GDPR	General Data Protection Regulation
GenAI	Generative Artificial Intelligence
GPT	Generative Pre-trained Transformer
HIPAA	Health Insurance Portability and Accountability Act
ICD	International Classification of Diseases
ICL	In-context Learning
LLaMA	Large Language Model Meta AI
LLaVA	Large Language and Vision Assistant
LLM	Large Language Model
LSTM	Long Short-Term Memory
QLoRA	Quantized Low-Ranked Adaptation
RBA	Risks, Benefits, and Alternatives
ROUGE	Recall-Oriented Understudy for Gisting Evaluation
SOAP	Subjective, Objective, Assessment, and Plan
WHO	World Health Organization

A. Taheri · A. Farhadi · A. Zamanifar (✉)
Department of Computer Engineering, Science and Research Branch, Islamic Azad University, Tehran, Iran
e-mail: alirezataheri@srbiau.ac.ir; amir.farhadi@srbiau.ac.ir; azamanifar@srbiau.ac.ir

A. Zamanifar, M. Faezipour (eds.), *Application of Generative AI in Healthcare Systems*, https://doi.org/10.1007/978-3-031-82963-5_4

1 Introduction

Generative artificial intelligence (GenAI) has made revolutionary changes across many fields. Beyond its well-known applications in conversational content generation, generative models are also used for domain adaptation [1], which involves transferring knowledge from a source domain to a target domain with different distributions [2, 3], text classification and sentiment analysis [4], feature extraction [5], data augmentation [6], translation [7], etc. Healthcare has also been significantly impacted by GenAI and its outstanding abilities in understanding and generation data. With the growing populations and the total number of people using healthcare systems around the world, the need for more efficient solutions to handle these cases has become more prominent. Generative AI language models, proved extraordinary skills in understanding and generating data, can revolutionize the way that our current healthcare systems work. Automating the documentation of clinical activities, provides countless opportunities for GenAI to make the hassling processes easier for medical personnel and patients. Utilizing generative tools benefits doctors and medical staff, as they will be allowed to spend less time on routine processes and focus more on care progress. Also, patients would be benefited by receiving quality care and spending more time with their physician [8, 9].

Due to the high complexity and multifaceted nature of natural languages, tasks that involve such data, were usually executed by humans. With rapid development of generative models and the active research in this field, these models are now capable of understanding natural language and the underlying relationship among words in text. Generative AI models are able to comprehend input text, and generate a corresponding answer that can include text, image or video. Text-based tasks are usually more common within the healthcare administrative support, that require a model that can read, understand, and analyze text, then output the desired information. On the other hand, for gathering information from multiple sources, or outputting data in different forms, there is limited functionality for unimodal models. Therefore, to better integrate into the workflow, multimodal systems are more preferable [10]. These models can be very useful in helping administrative staff by automating tasks, increasing efficiency and providing insight. There are a variety of tasks that can leverage such models ranging from note-taking, document management, to medical coding, pre-authorization and real-time transcription.

Technological advancements in the healthcare industry have contributed to increased life expectancy and average age. Population growth has led to a higher demand for medical and clinical services, which resulted in building more hospitals, clinics and medical centers. However, in some places the newly built medical centers cannot keep up with the pace of population growth and need for healthcare services. The increasing number of visits for the emergency department of the United States has raised concerns about degradation of care quality, patient dissatisfaction, and rising medical staff exhaustion [11]. Many countries are now facing shortage of physicians and clinicians. In case of natural disasters or crisis, this issue might even turn into a bigger challenge.

Digitalizing healthcare related information such as patients' medical history, has many advantages over traditional paper-based data entry and storage. Access to a patient's medical history and all the relevant information can enable healthcare providers to make more informed decisions and deliver better-quality care. Electronic health records (EHR) have significantly reduced errors and benefited medical services, however, handling them usually leads to extra work and is time-consuming [12]. Many studies have been conducted on the effect of EHR system on well-being of healthcare providers, and it seems that it adversely affects their job-satisfaction and contributes to burnout and chronic stress [13]. Thus, managing EHR can negatively influence patient care by consuming healthcare providers' time and reducing the quality of medical services. However, generative models have demonstrated a significant capacity to understand structured data, and can make good use of EHR by integrating into the healthcare system. These models are substantially beneficial for the medical staff and can alleviate workload and save more time for focusing on patients care. Leveraging these models in the field of clinical administration support, enables physicians to allocate more time for patient care, treatment, monitoring or other areas that might need more attention. A seamless integration of GenAI into the healthcare system can provide clinicians with patient clinical histories, streamline document review, and rapidly extract necessary data, thereby optimizing workflows and mitigating administrative burdens through reduced manual workload [14, 15]. Most AI systems can directly access EHRs to facilitate data entry and retrieval, which enhances the efficiency of healthcare delivery [16].

In healthcare areas like administrative support are more suitable for automation as they have lower-risk compared to diagnosis and treatment [17] and can substantially reduce the cost of care. GenAI models appear particularly promising in this field [18]. Not only do AI models positively affect clinician well-being, but also reduce administrative costs by minimizing manual labor and potential errors [19, 20]. Routine clerical tasks, such as scheduling meetings and efficiently allocating time to appointments, can also benefit from automation [21]. Patients can also benefit from patient-friendly documentation and notes, as well as increased time with clinicians and personalized attention.

General-purpose AI, such as ChatGPT, Gemini, or Microsoft Copilot have demonstrated excellent abilities in various tasks including NLP and Computer Vision. These models that are mostly conversational, have been used in various studies and their potential in clinical tasks is evaluated. However, more specialized generative models are required to be designed and trained on specific data to gain more understanding of clinical tasks. There are generalist medical models [22] that are trained on medical data and can be used to streamline many clinical workflows. These medical GenAI models might achieve better results compared to general-purpose ones, and address a wide range of tasks, including LLaVA-Med and Med-PaLM. On the other hand, there are more specific models that are developed and focused on performing a particular task within the healthcare field. These expert GenAI models seem more promising in facilitating different procedures as they are trained and designed to accomplish a constrained set of objectives. Take Med-Gemini [23] as an example, which is a family of models built on top of Gemini, a powerful general purpose AI foundation. Unlike generalist medical AI, these models are more application based and target specific specialties.

Despite excellent abilities in understanding and analyzing data, there is still a lot of areas that GenAI needs to get better at. As long as there are challenges such as hallucination, bias and other limitations, physicians and patients might not totally trust in these systems. To address the risks of using GenAI in healthcare, more research is required to mitigate the problems and issues inherent in generative models. The various limitations and risks to use GenAI in healthcare overlap in different administrative applications, hence, they will be discussed in a separate section.

In this chapter we aim to review the GenAI applications in administrative support. Generative models and their implementation in healthcare is still in early years of development. However, there are invaluable studies regarding building new models or innovative methods to use the existing GenAI systems. We present several models and approaches that each tried to take a step forward in facilitating medical workflows and increase quality of patient care. The rest of this chapter is presented in the following sections: Section 2 explores different types that GenAI can be integrated into healthcare systems. Section 3 elaborates on the different applications and areas in which generative models can be utilized to improve processes. Section 4 discusses some of the risks, challenges, and limitations associated with GenAI exploitation for administrative purposes. Finally, we conclude this chapter in Sect. 5.

2 Integration and Deployment

There are various ways in which GenAI systems can be integrated into the existing healthcare infrastructure. By embedding these models into the healthcare workspace, medical centers can enjoy efficiency, accuracy and patient-centric care. One approach is to deploy GenAI in the background as an ambient AI system. In this way, they can be used as digital medical scribes, by listening to the conversation between patients and providers. Automatic transcription is very helpful in reducing documentation burden and have the whole dialogue documented in real-time. Furthermore, GenAI can analyze the final document, summarize it, and highlight patient symptoms or other important sections as the doctor prefers. Additionally, GenAI can be integrated into the tools used by medical staff. This allows clinicians to leverage the model's capabilities in their everyday tasks. For instance, GenAI can assist in generating different documents, medical coding and billing, patient data extraction, EHR management, etc. Combining ambient AI note generation and EHR systems can transform healthcare workflows and facilitate medical data entry tasks. Seamlessly integrating real-time transcription, extracted medical information, and AI-generated drafts into the patients' medical records can help clinicians access a comprehensive view of medical records. This integration streamlines workflows and reduces documentation errors. Additionally, ambient AI can enhance EHR functionality by suggesting relevant information and flagging potential inconsistencies which ultimately improves patient care and service quality.

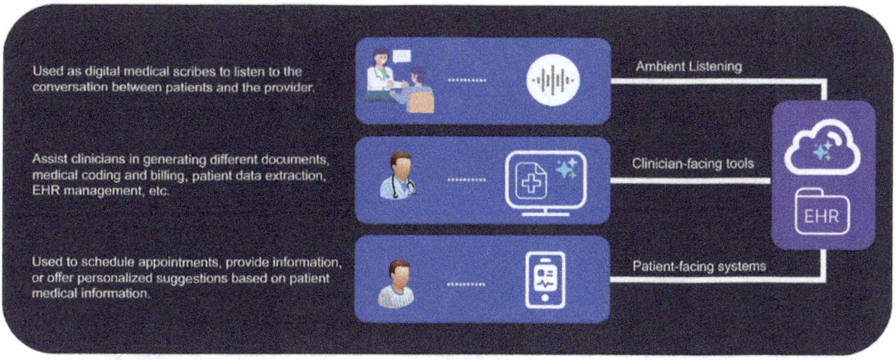

Fig. 1 Overview of the potential GenAI integration types for healthcare administrative support

Patients can also benefit from GenAI through patient-facing systems. These AI-powered systems can be used to schedule appointments, provide information, or offer personalized suggestions based on patient medical information. Patient portals can be enhanced with GenAI to deliver simplified clinical notes, which are usually filled with complex medical terminology, or answer to their basic questions about doctor availability, or certain processes and paperwork. Figure 1 provides an overview of the discussed integration types within the healthcare system.

3 Applications

Given that clinical staff spend a large portion of their time on administrative tasks such as managing patient medical records, clinical documentation, and paperwork, improving efficiency in these areas will have a significant impact on their job satisfaction, care quality, and error reduction [24]. Figure 2 represents different applications of GenAI in healthcare administrative support.

3.1 Medical Language Simplification

When the important steps of diagnosis and trials are over, it is time to transfer the information to other sections and the patient. Medical language mostly contains technical terminology and abbreviations that are specialized and complex. It is of vital importance for the patient to understand their doctor to be able to follow treatment plans and medication schedules in order to act accordingly. By interpreting clinical notes, patients can easily access information about their health and current conditions. Automating this process will save tremendous amount of time for clinicians and help patients grasp their current situation. GenAI can overcome this

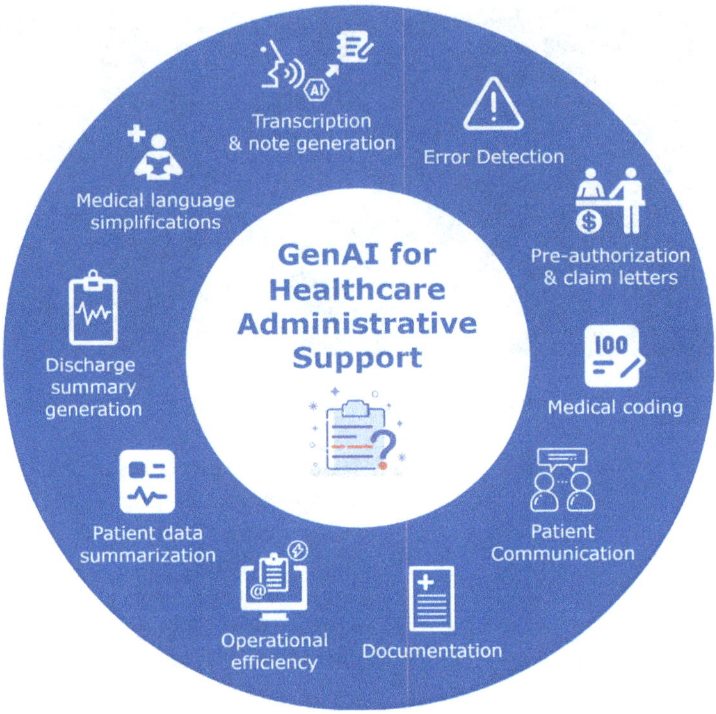

Fig. 2 Applications of GenAI in healthcare administrative support

challenging task by converting notes, trial results, treatments plans or any other medical document to a language that is easier for patients to understand. With the simplified documents, patients can be actively involved the process and enhance the experience and the results. Discharge summaries as an example, must be readily accessible for patients on demand. Doximity GPT as an example, can translate medical text to multiple languages and adjust the readability level to adapt to diverse audiences.

Various approaches have been proposed for generating simplified medical text, such as using language models [25] or ontologies [26]. Generative language models seem very helpful for this task as they possess the ability to grasp the meaning of complex medical notes and producing simplified versions with excellent grammar. Zaretsky et al. [27] used GPT-4 [28] to generate patient-friendly versions of discharge summaries. Prompt engineering and few-shot learning were used to reach the best results. They invited physicians to evaluate the generated discharge summaries. Generative AI proved useful in this study by improving readability and understandability for patients. They managed to reduce the reading level of the original discharge summaries from 11th grade to 6-seventh grade to make them more understandable by the general public.

Radiology reports are rich sources of information about current situation of the patient. They contain experts' opinions and interpretations from a wide variety of medical images. Understanding these notes can reduce the patient's anxiety and encourage them to follow treatment plans with more confidence [29]. Jeblick et al. [30] exploited ChatGPT to simplify radiology notes by prompting it to make the text understandable to a child. Although there were some incorrect statements or missed medical information, the generated reports were mostly correct, as voted by radiologists. Joseph et al. [31] used several generative models to evaluate their multilingual text simplification dataset. They tried zero-shot prompting on GPT-3 for both English to English and English to other languages. In monolingual experiments, they used Google Translate API to translate the results into the desired languages. Fine-tuned versions of T5 and Flan-T5 were also used to compare their performance. Results suggested that while GPT-3 generated fluent simplified text for English, it produced poor translation for other languages. Unlike fine-tuned T5, Flan-T5 failed to perform a decent job in simplifying while maintaining good grammar.

Lyu et al. [29] investigated the ability of ChatGPT to translate radiology reports into understandable notes for patients without any medical background. The length of a report contributes to the overall understandability of the document. The results suggested that ChatGPT tends to produce simplified documents with fewer words than the original versions. It also proved effective in replacing complex medical terminology with simple words to define them. This generative model showed great ability in integrating information from numerous experiments into simple sentences. There were a few cases of missing information which makes human supervision necessary. However, being able to automate most of the work is still very impressive and represents areas for improvement.

Tepe et al. [32] tried to simplify medical language to reduce the anxiety of patients after they receive their radiology report and before discussing them with their doctor. They compared the performance of Google Bard (now Gemini), Microsoft Copilot, and ChatGPT-4 in simplifying radiology reports, providing suggestions, and classifying severity of the conditions. Bard achieved superior results compared to other language models in terms of simplifying complex medical language in the reports, and lowering readability scores to eighth grade level. All models provided suggestions with high understandability with ChatGPT-4 achieving superior scores. In urgency detection, all models tend to stay on the safe side and classify most of the reports as emergencies in spite of the results being closer to normal.

3.2 Clinical Documentation

Clinical notes mostly contain patient visits, medical diagnoses, treatment strategies, and results. The adoption of EHR in healthcare organizations has brought many benefits for the patients and the system as a whole. Besides all these advantages, though, it proved to be a major contributor to clinicians' burnout and emotional exhaustion. This is sometimes referred to as clerical burden and has been detrimental to the overall job satisfaction and experience for medical staff. Many studies have been conducted to inspect the relationship between physician exhaustion and clinical documentation [13, 33]. Despite all the efforts for reducing the documentation burden supported by different organizations such as the American Medical Association, it is still one of the main contributors to the physician burnout and lower efficiency [33]. This issue sometimes leads to shortening clinic schedules to have extra time for clerical tasks. Many primary care physicians feel that most administrative tasks do not require a trained physician [13].

One of the primary applications of generative models in healthcare is creating high-quality human-like text. This makes them particularly ideal for tasks like generating medical documents by analyzing data. Giorgi et al. [34] address the challenge of automatically transforming patient-doctor dialogue into medical notes. They chose GPT-4 and used In-context Learning (ICL) which involves providing examples within the prompt to help the model produce more relevant and accurate results. GPT-4 showed little sensitivity to variations in prompt phrasing, therefore, they preferred to keep the length of the prompts shorter and make the instructions brief and simple. They compared the cosine similarity between dialogues and notes in the train set and selected the most similar note as an in-context example. The results suggest that using a note as an example is more effective than providing note-dialogue pairs. Also, providing more examples in prompts has minor improvements over just using one example. Evaluation by expert physicians suggests that the generated notes using GPT-4 are equally preferred to human-written notes, which indicates strong potential for automated note creation. Biswas et al. [35] went a step ahead and instead of using a ready-to-use patient-clinician interaction, they used Automatic Speech Recognition (ASR) to transcribe dialogues. For their training set, they used YouTube videos on experimental therapy sessions, and transcribed them using OpenAI Whisper [36]. One important challenge of this task is speaker diarization, which is clustering speech by different speakers. To support speaker diarization, which is vital in clinical documentation, they took various approaches. They tried and used an enhanced version of Whisper which can perform speaker diarization, but did not obtain high-quality data for note creation. In another approach they used GPT-3.5 to classify statements spoken by the doctor and the patient. Subjective, Objective, Assessment, and plan (SOAP) and Behavior, Intervention, Response, and Plan (BIRP) are two common types of medical notes that help clinicians organize their thoughts and opinions. In this study they used GPT-3.5 Turbo, GPT-4 Turbo, Claude V3, Mixtral and Llama to generate medical notes in SOAP and BIRP structures. The importance of prompt engineering to enhance performance is investigated in this study. They obtained varying results using simple instructions explaining the task, and some models were not completely successful to include all relevant knowledge and lacked consistency. By using one-shot prompting and providing more details, they were able to produce notes with higher quality and in the right format. They used several techniques in order to achieve the best prompt, such as, trial and error with output analysis, separating the task into smaller subtasks, and combining outputs of different models to exploit the strengths of each one. GPT-4 achieved the highest performance in documenting clinical conversations using ROUGE-1 score, followed by Claude, Llama and Mixtral.

MedicalSum [37] is a transformer-based model that incorporates medical knowledge from an external source to provide summaries of medical conversations. The advantage of leveraging medical information in the process of summarization is that the model can capture key medical details. The encoder and decoder of MedicalSum use several self-attention layers to help the model focus on more important parts of the text, which leads it to create accurate medical documentation.

Writing informed consents is another type of clinical document that is necessary to patient care. These forms are provided before performing any surgery to inform the patient and their family about their medical decision. These documents contain information about risks, benefits, and alternatives (RBA) of the coming procedure, and are important for the patient to read carefully, understand and concur with their contents. Decker et al. [38] evaluated the ability of ChatGPT-3.5 for generating RBAs. They determined the readability level of sixth grade in the prompt and asked ChatGPT to explain the risks, benefits, and alternatives of a certain procedure. In a total number of 36 surgical procedures, 6 of the RBAs were generated by ChatGPT and the rest were documented by surgeons. The mean readability score of both types of generated documents was at college level, with the AI-generated documents being less complex than that of surgeons. In terms of accuracy, AI-generated RBAs were all accurate and compared to 3 inaccurate surgeon-generated documents. Therefore, the results suggest that using LLMs in informed consent documentation is effective in generating complete, accurate and simple RBAs. Decoder-only transformers are used for generating medical reports from medical images in a study by Yang et al. [39] to address the physician burnout problem. They used a vision encoder and an LLM to decode the data. The results represent that ChatGLM-6B effectively captures the writing style of the reports and helps to generate optimal reports. Regard [40] is a clinician-oriented AI assistant that can enhance patient care by saving time on documentation and note generation. Regard AI Copilot can write clinical notes based on patient-relevant information or by voice input. With EHR integration, this tool can generate draft documentation for clinician review and seamlessly incorporate them into patient's medical record, which helps in streamlining the documentation process and reducing burden. Banner Health has integrated Regard's AI-powered tool across its 33 hospitals to streamline clinical documentation, alleviate administrative tasks, and improve patient care [41].

3.3 *Enhancing Operational Efficiency*

Generative models have exceptional abilities in handling everyday tasks that usually need little or no medical background proficiency. There are many common tools that administrative staff deal with almost every day for paperwork, scheduling appointments or meetings, documentation, etc. Influential companies that possess a large portion of the market with their various software products, can use the potential of GenAI to empower their tools and make the clerical workflow more efficient. In this regard Microsoft and Google have taken their GenAI models to a higher level by optimizing activities through common software programs such as Office 365 [42] or the entire Google Workspace. Copilot and Gemini [43] now enable users to work more efficiently by using the normal conversational chatbots or integrating into software programs to make scheduling appointments, sending and responding to emails, meeting management and summary generation, and many more easier [44]. Additionally, during international medical collaborations or meetings, GenAI can boost performance and maximize efficiency by providing real-time language translation. This can lead to enhanced collaboration and results [45].

Traditionally, all appointments and visits are manually handled by medical staff. Refilling a prescription involves obtaining additional medication to continue a prescribed treatment. Nurses spend a big portion of their time performing administrative tasks such as setting appointments and refilling prescriptions in addition to documentation and patient records management [45]. Generative AI can access appointment records, meeting lists, and in-office time for physicians and prioritize patients to set appointments. After putting their information, patients can also see the available time offered by the medical center to pick their preferred time slot. GenAI can also handle canceling appointments by rescheduling the required ones to help optimize their working hours, and more available face time for patients [46].

3.4 Discharge Summary Generation

Once a patient is discharged from a medical center, physicians create a comprehensive discharge summary, mentioning the patient's hospitalization and treatment. This document will then be attached to the medical records of the patient, accessible for future uses. Exploiting GenAI in automatically writing discharge summaries can reduce junior doctors' exhaustion and administration burden who are often responsible to perform this task [47]. Hartman et al. [48] used a fine-tuned version of BART to produce hospital course section of discharge summaries, which includes information about treatment progress from admission to discharge. They separated the original dataset into three sections including: patient history, daily treatment updates, and post-discharge follow-up details. To address the problem of hallucination and improve factuality, they employed constrained beam search. While this approach slightly lowered ROUGE score, it effectively reduced error rates within the sentences. Their model achieved high readability in the automatically generated summaries and obtained 62% quality standards of care, compared to 91% of that of physicians.

ChatGPT is also used to write discharge summaries using patient information in a study by Clough et al. [47]. They added the output structure and template in the prompt and asked ChatGPT to write a discharge summary based on the clinical note provided. A few junior doctors were also asked to write discharge summaries. All the generated summaries by ChatGPT were reviewed and considered acceptable by the general practitioners. The interesting point is that the AI-generated summaries were hardly distinguishable from that of junior doctors with only 60% accuracy in detection. Thereby, it represents the ability of LLMs in generating human-like text with high accuracy.

Van Veen et al. [49] conducted a study to assess the effectiveness of various LLMs in medical summarization. They selected 8 models including FLAN-T5, FLAN-UL2, Alpaca, Med-Alpaca, Vicuna, Llama-2, and versions 3.5 and 4 of GPT. In context learning (ICL) and QLoRA were used as two types of adaptation. Using only one example in ICL resulted in worse performance than QLoRA. On the other hand, by bringing as many examples as possible to fit in the prompt, it was shown that ICL outperforms QLoRA across various LLMs. The best performing model was GPT-4 with more complete and accurate summaries than that of human medical expert-generated summaries. GPT-4 was able to mostly correctly identify the relevant information from the input. Interestingly, the likelihood and impact of medical harm for human-generated summaries were higher compared to those of GPT-4. As the results show higher scores of completeness and correctness, LLMs can have a bright future in helping clinicians with summarization.

In a study conducted by Rosenberg et al. [9] AI-generated discharge summaries were compared to physician-generated summaries. A junior orthopedic surgeon and a senior orthopedic surgery resident were asked to write two different discharge documents. The discharge summary includes a detailed summary of the patient's hospital stay, diagnosis, history of the present illness, procedures, clinical summary and discharge guidelines. On the other hand, discharge letter is a simplified summary that is delivered to the patient. ChatGPT-4 is used to automatically generate both discharge documents for all cases using a same prompt. Both human- and machine-generated documents were evaluated by an expert team of orthopedic surgeons and residents. The results reveal that both types of generated summaries are acceptable and have similar quality. There were a few hallucination occurrences that show the importance of post-modifications. Overall, ChatGPT proved able to generate discharge summaries 10 times faster than human writers with almost similar quality.

3.5 Transcription and Note Creation

In a patient visit, a substantial amount of data is created which includes lab test requests, physical examination, patient history, alongside other notes and reports. The processes of taking notes, inputting into the EHR system, and maintaining records are time-consuming and prone to errors. Clinicians may choose to enter information into the computer during the patient visit or use a paper-based approach and digitize the data later. Both methods involve burdensome documentation and data entry, which might negatively impact the clinician and patient satisfaction. This issue can be addressed using ASR systems that can listen to conversations and automatically convert them into structured records [50]. There are several important and challenging tasks that are required for generative models to be able to listen to patient-doctor conversations and fill out forms, document, or summarize the content. First, it needs to convert speech into text, then comprehend and analyze text to extract key points and details. Finally, it generates the desired output in any format like SOAP or BIRP, or simple raw summaries. To make this happen, first the patient-clinician interaction needs to be recorded into audio files, then by applying ASR and diarization, each side's speech will be converted to text for the rest of the process. LLMs are trained on large amounts of text, therefore, are capable of understanding words and their relationships in documents. This ability makes these models comprehend the transcribed conversation and extract key points and important information related to the subject. Once the knowledge about the interaction is gathered, it is time to put it into the desired format. This stage can be done through prompting the model to produce a certain type of document with specific details and sections [45].

In the context of medical note generation, Adedeji and colleagues [51] used LLMs to improve the accuracy of ASR systems in medical transcription. They picked Gemini, GPT-4, LLaMA, Claude, and Text Bison to enhance the accuracy of Deepgram's Nova, Sonix, Amazon Transcribe Medical, OpenAI Whisper, and Google Cloud's Chirp and Medical Conversation model (GCMC). They utilized zero-shot and chain-of-thought prompting to correct transcription errors and diarize the conversation. One issue regarding the output of LLMs is keeping the integrity of the requested format that these models deviate from it from time to time. Therefore, regex-based post processing is used to extract the desired information from the output of LLMs. A comprehensive set of experiments was conducted that demonstrates the LLMs' ability to reduce error rates and improve diarization of the ASR generated transcriptions.

DAX Copilot by Nuance [16] is an AI-driven system that automates and improves clinical documentation by accurately capturing patient encounters in real-time. By using a secure mobile application that increases mobility, healthcare providers can have natural conversations with patients and their families without the distraction of manual documentation. This ambient AI technology allows clinicians to focus more on patient care rather than data entry. This GenAI is trained on over ten million encounters, and transforms spoken interactions into accurate clinical summaries that is accessible on both the mobile app and the Dragon Medical One platform for clinicians to review or modify. Dragon Medical One integrates with many EHR systems which helps enhancing overall clinical efficiency. This tool aims to reduce manual work by proposing many features like automatic punctuation insertion and voice commands. Nuance is currently deploying DAX Copilot in various medical centers in partnership with healthcare systems and hospitals, including Northwestern Medicine [52], Providence health and services [53], WellSpan Health [54], Intermountain health [55], etc.

Suki [56] is another AI healthcare solution that offers ASR and an assistant to automate clinical note creation and minimize administrative burden. It supports many languages and specialties and allows clinicians to dictate notes, or it can listen ambiently to patient encounters to generate clinical notes. Suki also helps in diagnostic coding and real-time information retrieval, making documentation even less time-consuming. EHR integration ensures data consistency and seamless data flow between the AI assistant and EHR systems, which reduces the need for data re-entry. Suki has partnered with a number of community health centers to implement its AI-powered scribe technology, enhancing clinical documentation efficiency and reducing administrative burden [57].

PhenoPad, proposed by Wang et al. [50] addressed several challenges faced by clinicians in hospitals. As the results of a survey of physicians at the Hospital for Sick Children in Toronto, they reported that EHR systems made it hard for clinicians to give patients their full attention while taking notes, mostly because they often had to look down at their computers or have their hands occupied during examinations. They also found it difficult to document physical examinations and observations without additional devices. Transferring information from external medical devices into the EHR system is also a time-consuming process. PhenoPad provides a note-taking interface that allows clinicians to write notes on a tablet or use speech recognition. Numerous sessions conducted in different sections of the hospital demonstrated that this system effectively enhanced the medical workflows and reduce clinical note-taking burden.

3.6 Patient Communication

One of the administration burdens for clinicians is the massive number of messages from patients in their inbox. Garcia et al. [58] conducted a pilot quality improvement project at Stanford Health Care with the enrollment of medical staff from different divisions. They sorted out incoming messages from patients into distinct categories including general, results, medication, and paperwork. They inputted patient messages and medical information along with their latest clinical note to GPT-4 and provided personnel with options to review and use the draft or start writing a response from scratch. Although there was not considerable time saving, their research is remarkable in many aspects. In spite of using the general GPT-4 model with no fine-tuning or background specific medical knowledge, the generated draft responses could reduce clinicians' exhaustion and administrative burden. Additionally, using more documents and information for generating each message, could probably help GPT-4 produce better responses. The fact that it needed minimal staff preparation for integrating this LLM into the EHR system, makes it suitable for future implementation on a larger scale.

In order to make generative models ready to deploy, we need to make sure that they meet certain requirements such as minimum evaluation scores. To enhance patient experience, the summarized information can be accessible for them via mobile and web applications. Dependent on the policies or user preferences, generated simplified summaries can be presented in raw format or in certain templates and structures [45]. The presence of a verified medical chat bot can also help reduce workload by answering any raised questions about different parts of the shown document.

Ellen AI [59] is a text-to-voice tool that complements GenAI models by transforming written information into clear spoken content. This tool can significantly enhance patient communication by providing voice interaction layer between the backbone GenAI (e.g. ChatGPT) and the patient. Healthcare providers can leverage this technology to deliver vital information such as medical instructions, discharge summaries, or any educational material to patients who prefer audio formats or those with visual impairments. Utilizing this tool can effectively improve overall patient care.

3.7 Patient Data Summarization

Medical doctors always need to be updated with the latest information of their patients. They need to be aware of symptoms, prior visits and treatments, and their medical history to make an informed decision. Facing a lot of documents and extract important points poses a risk of burnout. With much of the information available electronically, generative models can read through all the documents, understand the key points and provide a summary of the whole information in brief sections highlighting the most important matters to consider. These summaries can contain key medical details including diagnosis and treatment plans or can just remind a family physician of their patient's current situation [46]. Providing summaries of patient medical history and current conditions has countless potentials in every stage of medical operations by providing valuable insights about the relationship between different aspects and making suggestions.

One big advantage of the success of general language models can be attributed to their massive scale and large numbers of parameters, in addition to the vast amounts of training material. Yang et al. [60] proposed GatorTron to investigate the extent of the dataset and model scale on the performance of the language models in the healthcare domain. Unlike previous studies that usually set the number of parameters on a scale of millions, GatorTron has 8.9 billion parameters and is trained on more than 90 billion words to enhance the performance. The results suggest that scaling up the parameters and training dataset size, has significant improvement on more complex clinical tasks such as natural language inference and question answering, but less improvement for simpler ones including clinical concept extraction. This large-scale medical language model is promising in streamlining workflows in various sections in healthcare. GatorTron can make unstructured EHR management easier for clinicians, and improve accuracy and prevent errors. It demonstrates the potential of GenAI and LLMs in the field of healthcare to automate administrative tasks such as medical documentation and coding in EHR systems and alleviate the heavy burden on clinicians [61].

Almanac Copilot [62] is developed by Cyril et al. to facilitate clinical workflows and streamline administrative tasks. This framework helps clinicians by assisting them in EHR-related tasks such as navigating complex EHR systems, data entry and manipulation. They provided the model with access to various tools such as a browser, calculators, and the EHR system itself. To level up the LLM's ability, it can have access to all the tools in order to make a comprehensive decision regarding incoming commands through prompts.

3.8 Medical Coding

Various types of clinical diagnosis and the discovery of new diseases over time require a clear and standardized system to identify and track diseases over time and across different places. Clinical notes in medical records are written in free-form text, which requires a unified system for classifying them. Potential applications of such systems include tracking care progress, consistent documentation and organization, service analysis, data sharing and research, health resource planning, medical billing, and reimbursement. International Classification of Diseases (ICD), established by the World Health Organization (WHO), has been a main categorization system for medical coding worldwide [63]. The 11th version of ICD (ICD-11), adopted in May 2019, is more extensive than the earlier versions and came into effect in January 2022 [64]. Despite its myriad benefits, manual ICD coding is labor-intensive and time-consuming. It requires comprehensive knowledge about the ICD system and an understanding of clinical notes. Hence, automating medical coding has been an interesting subject in NLP and can also be addressed by GenAI. Not only can automated medical coding streamline the coding process and decrease the administrative burden, but also it can potentially increase accuracy and reduce error rates. In spite of having internal and external auditors, errors still occur and inaccurate coding can cause significant financial consequences [65].

Soroush et al. evaluated the performance of famous general LLMs including Gemini Pro, Llama2-70b in detecting medical codes given the descriptions. This study aimed to investigate the extent of accuracy of LLMs in their base form with no advanced prompt engineering, fine-tuning or any additional module or tool. The results demonstrate that these models are poor medical coders and none of them could surpass 50% accuracy in any dataset. The important implication of this study is that we cannot expect superior performance from general LLMs without fine-tuning or external knowledge in highly specialized fields. The most important issues that make the task of medical coding challenging for these models include explainability, data scarcity for specific codes, higher recall and low precision, large label space, and long sequences [66, 67].

There have been various approaches to medical coding including rule-based and deep learning methods. Li et al. [67] explored a multi-agent system for automatically detecting medical codes using GPT-4. This system simulates real-world human behavior in ICD coding. It consists of agents including a patient, a physician, a coder, a reviewer and an adjuster that each use an instance of LLM to imitate the interaction. After the physician agent visits the patient, the coder assigns the codes according to the medical notes. After the reviewer agent reviews the codes, the physician and patient will view the results and if they disagree, the adjuster agent makes the decision. They used SOAP structure to mitigate the hallucination problem of LLMs and increase accuracy. An external knowledge base of code descriptions is also added to boost the performance of the models. The results show that the presented approach can effectively enhance the performance of medical coding compared to the baselines.

Yang et al. [66] proposed LLM-codex, a hybrid method based on LLMs to accurately automate the medical coding procedure. Their approach uses GPT-4 to first identify ICD codes within a document. The prompt consists of the clinical note in addition to a predefined set of ICD codes for the LLM to assign to each document. After a list of possible codes is provided, in the next step, they feed this again to the LLM and ask it to assign each sentence one or more of the detected ICD codes. Then a list of sentences and their corresponding ICD codes are obtained as evidence. The final stage contains an LSTM model to predict which of the provided pairs of evidence sentences and ICD codes are correct based on the document-level real labels. The verifier model leverages the high recall of the LLM output and high precision of the expert medical coder. The results suggest that this two-stage approach could improve the precision-recall balance and f1-score compared to the baseline models.

Corti's Code Automate [68] can significantly reduce workload of providers by reducing a lot of hours of administrative tasks which will save a significant amount of money and resources. Once a clinical documentation is done, Corti reads it and identifies the accurate medical codes. This AI-assistant supports many coding systems such as ICD-10 and Current Procedural Terminology (CPT), and can effectively reduce claim denial rates.

3.9 Error Detection

With the growing number of patient visits, documentation, and the related paperwork regarding handling different aspects of healthcare services, the increase in the number of errors embodied within the information will rise inevitably. The risk of having inconsistencies in medical information and wrong data entry can have costly or even fatal consequences. Text-based GenAI models are often used for grammatical and writing style correction, therefore, they seem promising in detecting and correcting errors in medical documents to prevent any mistaken record or document being submitted or used.

In a study conducted by Tung et al. [69] a comparison between the generated discharge summaries written by generative models and junior clinicians is presented. Junior doctors are usually tasked with labor-intensive and time-consuming documentation to ensure consistent care. In this study, GPT-4 was able to provide clinicians with holistic summaries that were mostly lengthier than that of clinicians. The clinicians made 1.7 grammatical mistakes per letter. In contrast, the discharge summaries generated by GPT-4 contained no instances of any grammatical error which demonstrates its ability in generating documents with high readability.

Yakovchuk et al. [70] in an attempt to digitalize medical prescriptions, used LLMs as an additional layer of error detection. They converted paper prescriptions to text using a handwriting recognition module. ChatGPT was used to analyze the generated text, recognize and correct any possible errors in it. The results show that GenAI can detect grammatical errors of the recognition module along with mistakes made by the clinician in writing the prescription.

In addition to writing mistakes, LLMs can be used as a safeguard within the EHR system to identify potential oversight in patient medical records. These models offer an additional layer of review which helps in preventing errors stemming from mistakes in diagnosis and medication [46]. Corti detects medical coding inaccuracies and insufficient documentation, highlights potential documentation deficiencies, and identifies under- and over-coding to enhance overall efficiency and prevent any errors before billing.

3.10 Pre-authorization and Claim Letters

Part of patient satisfaction is possible through fast processing of paperwork before, during and after discharge. By resolving insurance claims and pre-authorization, patients can experience a better service during their hospitalization. Pre-authorization refers to the process by which insurance companies decide whether to approve or deny coverage for particular medical treatments, procedures, or medication when a patient requires them. It is designed to control costs, while it is usually time-consuming for healthcare providers. Additionally, healthcare payers or insurance companies dedicate substantial time for reviewing prior-authorization requests. This administrative burden is perceived by clinicians as it delays timely treatment. Automating pre-authorization accelerates data flow and will save a considerable amount of time that can be used to handle challenging cases and improve care quality [71]. Fully automating this task can lower the impact of increase in claim requests, however, a semi-automated process will also help in reducing manual labor. GenAI can help gather the required information with the help of the accessible tools and summarize them in desired formats to help make decisions faster with quick information access. Implementing such systems will require new regulations for safely transferring EHR [71].

GenAI can streamline insurance claims processing by automating the pipeline of claim assessment including document analysis and verification. This helps reducing errors and time spent on processing the claims, which enhances patient satisfaction through faster claim resolution [46, 72]. In a collaboration of OpenAI and Doximity, a medical AI assistant is built to help clinicians with various administrative tasks to reduce burden and increase their time for patient care. Doximity GPT is a writing assistant that uses GPT-4 to write pre-authorization and insurance appeal letters to streamline workflows.

Jiang et al. [73] proposed NYUTron, a medical LLM that is capable of performing various clinical tasks including insurance denial prediction on admission. The target of this model in this task is to predict whether the insurance company accepts or denies the submitted claim upon admission. This model uses available information within the admission or discharge notes to predict the denial of the claim. NYUTron could achieve better performance compared to traditional models and showed promise as a clinical assistant. Additionally, GenAI can be employed for fraudulent claim detection. Although previous studies have successfully utilized BERT-based methods [74] for this task, GenAI can also be used to identify patterns associated with fraudulent claims and notify for investigation [72].

4 Challenges, Limitations and Potential Risks

There are numerous benefits to using GenAI to overcome various challenges and difficulties in healthcare. The aim of using GenAI in administrative support is to streamline labor-intensive and heavy workflows that hinder clinicians to provide quality care for patients. Using LLMs in other fields and industries might be totally fine for speeding up processes with minimum supervision. However, when it comes to healthcare, the life and well-being of people is at stake which makes the safety and sensitivity of the automation more important. Medical industry will enjoy automation through the use of GenAI, as long as it complies with certain rules and constraints to make it safe. Besides safety, accountability and explainability are crucial in order to apply GenAI to medical workflows. Data integrity, confidentiality, and accessibility are other important factors in implementing these systems. The administrative applications that are previously mentioned can be facilitated by using the proposed approaches by researchers. Nonetheless, it is still vital to have human supervision to assess the correctness and the output of the models. While these models made breakthroughs in understanding and analyzing sequential data, their reliability remains imperfect, particularly when considering the potential risks of errors in healthcare. Therefore, it is of vital importance to know the possible limitations and risks associated with these models before starting to integrate them into the field. Knowing the challenges of incorporating GenAI can lead to improvements and optimization, and also making informed decisions whether and how to utilize these models to make the most out of them.

Here we review a number of challenges and risks that might adversely affect applying GenAI to the mentioned tasks as represented in Fig. 3. The followings are related to the administrative applications of GenAI and do not include other possible risks in other fields, such as plagiarism in medical research. Addressing these shortcomings will help increasing the trust of users in these systems, which is critical for the adoption of GenAI [75].

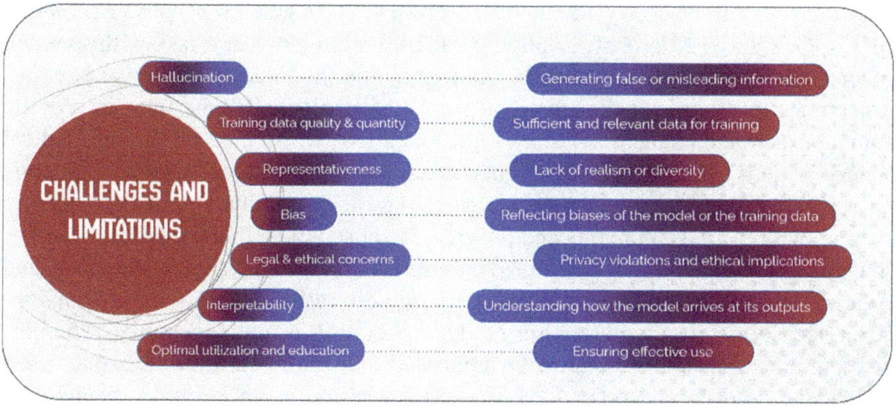

Fig. 3 Challenges and limitations of GenAI in healthcare administration support

4.1 Hallucination

LLMs exhibit outstanding ability in generating natural, persuasive, and coherent responses, which makes it hard to identify errors and misinformation. LLM hallucinations occur when the generated content is not reliable, misleading, and not grounded in reality. GenAI models are powerful enough to generate seemingly correct data with high confidence that is difficult to detect [76]. The sensitivity of the field of healthcare, makes this problem even more worthy of notice as errors have greater consequences. Hallucinations that are embedded among the facts, are more concerning when patients face them. Patients are more vulnerable to erroneous content as they do not possess the knowledge of an expert like a clinician to detect and act upon mistakes. Rarity does not lower the risk of hallucination in medical applications, as several studies found instances of fabrication in the generated output by LLMs [9]. Hallucination can always occur in different tasks and many studies acknowledge their existence as known hallucinations, and others propose ideas to mitigate them [48]. Therefore, complete dependence on generative models even the ones that seem so powerful, is still unwarranted.

4.2 Training Data Quality and Quantity

Good performing GenAI models are very big in scale of their parameters and also require a large number of training data. Current state-of-the-art LLMs like GPT-4 are trained on vast amounts of data that make them able to grasp the natural language complexity and the relationship among the words. However, providing this massive body of corpus to train the model on, can be found challenging. The quality of the data is critical as it determines the accuracy and reliability of the model. The training data needs to be balanced, cleaned, and be of high quality, which for very large datasets can be costly and labor-intensive [77]. In general purpose LLMs like GPT-4, Gemini, or Microsoft Copilot, it can be a relatively easier task with so much general text already available on the internet and in the databases of organizations. It becomes more of a challenge when the LLM is planned to be used in specific domains such as healthcare. There is not much real-world data of patient medical history or EHR available due to patients' privacy and regulations. Another challenge of exploiting GenAI in the domains that require expert skills is that they need to keep up with the developments and progress in those fields. In the medical industry, changes in standards like ICD or maybe treatment of certain diseases, diagnosis and policies are not rare. Using a GenAI to suggest old treatments or use an old-fashioned style for summarization or documentation is not acceptable. Thereby, these models constantly need to be upgraded and make sure they use the latest knowledge on different topics [78]. Coding guidelines as an example change over time in order to include more precise definition of diseases which need to be considered when developing automated medical coding systems. With a large number of disease codes, coding models require to take into account the less frequent codes, rare diagnoses for which there are not as many instances in the training data [79]. Keeping the models updated with the latest changes and discoveries in healthcare, and providing high quality data in massive scales, can be a challenge in front of researchers and implementors of these models. Undoubtedly, the cost of training GenAI on these massive data periodically in terms of providing enough processing power needs to be noted [10, 18].

4.3 Authenticity and Representativeness

Creating fair models requires training them with balanced datasets that reflects the diversity and variety of the real-world scenarios. Obtaining large amounts of training data in the field of healthcare is very challenging as there are strict regulations and rules concerning personal medical information. There need to be safeguards in place regarding making all the data unidentifiable and ensure that no personal information that can be traced back to an individual is released. This can lead to relatively smaller datasets compared to the ones that LLMs need to actually be capable of achieving decent performance. The more data available to GenAI models, the better they will be in understanding the field. Training data must be complete, diverse and representative of the different scenarios that the model will encounter in real-world [77]. By acquiring data that is vast enough to cover rare cases, the bias related to the dataset can be reduced and the final model will be more robust and accurate.

4.4 *Bias*

One of the advantages of exploiting AI in different tasks is that the opinion of the models is not subjective and influenced by personal beliefs or opinions, therefore, it can analyze and make decisions solely based on the original material and data it was exposed to. Nonetheless, the issue with bias does not end here, and bias can be related to either data or the model. The data on which the model is trained on might be discriminatory, biased towards certain concepts, or prefer something just because it has seen more information about it frequently during the training stage [80]. It is of vital importance to have more control over the data when training medical LLMs than general ones.

4.5 *Legal and Ethical Concerns*

Regulation and ethical issues include a vast array of challenges that need to be addressed before successfully deploying GenAI into medical systems. Privacy, comprehensive regulations, and humanistic issues are important concerns in developing medical generative models. Current studies are mostly conducted on publicly available datasets that do not reveal any individual identifiable information. Although in order to take a step forward or deploy these models in real-world scenarios, GenAI needs to access a lot of information about patients for training and inference. This does raise concerns about privacy and data security. To ensure patients that their information is safely protected and used, there should be stricter regulations regarding handling EHRs. In case of any data breach or misuse of data, there will be significant risks of identity theft and privacy violation [10]. With introducing new systems that can transfer, process or store data, the risk of compromising data confidentiality will increase. Also, there needs to be a verification of regulatory compliance of AI systems that can guarantee adhering to the latest laws and policies [10]. The Health Insurance Portability and Accountability Act in the United States protects patient personal health information (PHI), and GDPR safeguards personal information across the European Union. These legislations are two examples of such laws that can protect personal data to which AI systems must be compliant [45]. These regulations might even prohibit sharing models between medical centers in order to make sure no identifiable information is leaked [79]. There are strict regulations for software programs that handle patient information and help in decision making that are referred to as software as a medical device across the world [81]. A few commercial AI assistants such as Doximity GPT and Suki support regulations regarding handling PHI, and are fully HIPAA compliant to be trusted in medical workflow. Humanistic considerations are crucial for GenAI for making them pay attention to patient-physician relationship along with having compassion and empathy [82]. GenAI must be able to take respect and human emotions into consideration especially when facing patients with their questions, trial results, or simplified documentation.

4.6 Interpretability

Due to the black-box nature of LLMs, the source of the generated recommendations, summarization, or diagnosis can hardly be explained or interpreted. Although there are many studies targeting explainability, AI research was mainly focused on improving predictive power and generating spectacular content [83]. Knowing the source of the information and how the model arrives at its results might actually raise the healthcare workers' trust in using GenAI as an assistant as they can easily interpret the results and follow the chain that led to output. With low interpretability, pinpointing mistakes might be harder and users will have a hard time interpreting or understanding the output [77]. As the level of explainability rises, the role of clinicians as supervisors will be more straightforward and the collaboration of the AI system and the staff will be enhanced [10]. Explainability is crucial for GenAI as it involves regulations, ethical concerns, and trust in these models [83]. Using closed-source LLMs such as GPT-4, Gemini, or Claude might present several additional challenges. The proprietary nature of these models prevents direct access to the inner workings. These powerful LLMs are only accessible through API calls which allows limited customization and interpretability. This lack of flexibility, transparency and difficulty in understanding how these models arrive at their decisions hinder the ability to assess for potential biases, and reliable responses [84, 85].

4.7 Optimal Utilization and Education

GenAI models are very powerful and capable of performing a variety of tasks fluently and with high accuracy. However, unleashing this power requires knowledge and understanding of interacting with them. LLMs receive commands in natural language through prompts, and after reading and comprehending the request they generate the output. It is empirically and research-proven that how the request is written in the prompt directly affects the generated results. It is widely believed that using a comprehensive and accurate prompt to precisely address the need works decently well to achieve the best results possible. On the other hand, sometimes it does not make any significant difference and simpler prompts might actually produce good results too.

Providing users with GenAI will require educating them on how to state their commands and ask GenAI to produce the corresponding output. This allows them to make the most out of the model and utilize its potential. Prompt engineering becomes more important when the medical staff are provided with the model in a conversational manner that requires them to come up with the best prompt. Although

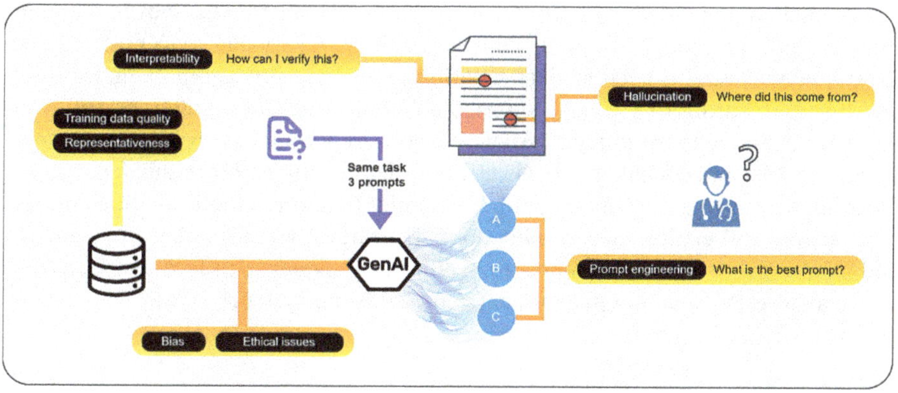

Fig. 4 Challenges and limitations of using GenAI in generating a document

in routine tasks that usually take place in the same situation, or the input comes from a determined source, the prompt engineering process can be comprehensively done before deployment and clinicians will be provided with the best performing prompt requiring only changing a few parameters.

GenAI can potentially augment staff capabilities or maybe displace some jobs dealing with routine tasks that are easily performed by these models with high quality. This requires a shift in training and educating clinical staff to help them better adapt to their new AI-related duties [10]. It is also worth noting that with the prevalence of AI in various fields, workers might gradually be more dependent on them to a degree that they lose their ability of performing those tasks on their own (Fig. 4).

5 Conclusion

The integration of generative models into healthcare administration offers numerous advantages for both clinicians and patients, and also benefits the medical system as a whole. By automating routine tasks, GenAI can alleviate workload on healthcare staff and allow them to focus more on the quality of patient care. Moreover, this increased time for patient interaction can also enhance patient communication and foster stronger patient-provider relationship. Additionally, GenAI can help reduce the administrative burden and lower pressure on medical staff, which improves physician well-being and overall job satisfaction. Furthermore, GenAI has the potential to improve efficiency and management within healthcare organizations and reduce operational costs.

It is crucial to acknowledge and address the challenges and limitations associated with implementing and integrating GenAI. The black-box nature of these models can make it difficult to understand how they arrive at their conclusions. The performance of GenAI heavily relies on the quality and quantity of training data, which can be challenging due to legal concerns. Additionally, unintended bias in the training data and the model can contribute to unfair decisions and inaccurate results. Ethical considerations such as data security and patient privacy must be carefully addressed. Ensuring that GenAI systems adhere to relevant regulations and standards is necessary to avoid legal issues. It is also important to consider the changes in current jobs and educate medical staff in order to fully embrace this technology. Ongoing research and development are essential to address the limitations of current models and explore new applications. By carefully considering these factors and adopting a responsible approach, healthcare providers can leverage GenAI to create a more efficient and patient-centered healthcare system.

References

1. Muffoletto M, et al. Combining generative modelling and semi-supervised domain adaptation for whole heart cardiovascular magnetic resonance angiography segmentation. J Cardiovasc Magn Reson. 2023;25(1):80.
2. Farhadi A, Sharifi A. Leveraging meta-learning to improve unsupervised domain adaptation. Comput J. 2024;67(5):1838–50.
3. Farhadi A, et al. Domain adaptation in reinforcement learning: a comprehensive and systematic study. J Zhejiang Univ Sci C. 2024;25:1446–65.
4. Krugmann JO, Hartmann J. Sentiment analysis in the age of generative AI. Cust Needs Solut. 2024;11(1):3.
5. Farhadi A, et al. Unsupervised domain adaptation for image classification based on deep neural networks. Intelligent Multimedia Proc Commun Syst (IMPCS). 2023;4(1):27–37.
6. Taheri A, Zamanifar A, Farhadi A. Enhancing aspect-based sentiment analysis using data augmentation based on back-translation. Int J Data Sci Anal. 2024:1–26.
7. Siu SC. Revolutionising translation with AI: unravelling neural machine translation and generative pre-trained large language models. In: New advances in translation technology: applications and pedagogy. Singapore: Springer; 2024. p. 29–54.
8. Loh E. ChatGPT and generative AI chatbots: challenges and opportunities for science, medicine and medical leaders. BMJ Leader. 2023;8:leader-2023-000797.
9. Rosenberg GS, et al. ChatGPT-4 generates orthopedic discharge documents faster than humans maintaining comparable quality: a pilot study of 6 cases. Acta Orthop. 2024;95:152.
10. Okonji OR, Yunusov K, Gordon B. Applications of generative AI in Healthcare: algorithmic, ethical, legal and societal considerations. arXiv. 2024. Preprint arXiv:2406.10632.
11. Moy AJ, et al. Understanding the perceived role of electronic health records and workflow fragmentation on clinician documentation burden in emergency departments. J Am Med Inform Assoc. 2023;30(5):797–808.
12. Wachter RM, Brynjolfsson E. Will generative artificial intelligence deliver on its promise in health care? JAMA. 2024;331(1):65–9.
13. Budd J. Burnout related to electronic health record use in primary care. J Prim Care Community Health. 2023;14:21501319231166921.
14. DiGiorgio AM, Ehrenfeld JM. Artificial intelligence in medicine & ChatGPT: de-tether the physician. J Med Syst. 2023;47(1):32.
15. Ustymenko S, Phadke A. Promise and challenges of generative AI in healthcare information systems. In: Proceedings of the 2024 ACM southeast conference 2024.
16. The new era of AI copilots for healthcare. [cited 13 August 2024]; Available from: https://www.nuance.com/healthcare/campaign/learn-more/dax-copilot.html.

17. Bhasker S, et al. Tackling healthcare's biggest burdens with generative AI. McKinsey & Company; United States. 2023. p. 10.
18. Etli D. Generative AI and patient care: a systematic review examining applications, limitations, and future directions for ChatGPT in healthcare. J Qual Health Care Econ. 2024:7.
19. Prabhod KJ. The role of artificial intelligence in reducing healthcare costs and improving operational efficiency. Q J Emerg Technol Innov. 2024;9(2):47–59.
20. Singh JP. The impacts and challenges of generative artificial intelligence in medical education, clinical diagnostics, administrative efficiency, and data generation. Int J Appl Health Care Anal. 2023;8(5):37–46.
21. Johnson B. Revolutionizing healthcare with generative AI. BMH Med J. ISSN 2348–392X. 2024;11(2):31–4.
22. Moor M, et al. Foundation models for generalist medical artificial intelligence. Nature. 2023;616(7956):259–65.
23. Saab K, et al. Capabilities of gemini models in medicine. arXiv. 2024. Preprint arXiv:2404.18416.
24. Tursunbayeva A, Renkema M. Artificial intelligence in health-care: implications for the job design of healthcare professionals. Asia Pac J Hum Resour. 2023;61(4):845–87.
25. Lu J, et al. Napss: paragraph-level medical text simplification via narrative prompting and sentence-matching summarization. arXiv. 2023. Preprint arXiv:2302.05574.
26. Moramarco F, et al. Towards more patient friendly clinical notes through language models and ontologies. In: AMIA annual symposium proceedings. American Medical Informatics Association; 2021.
27. Zaretsky J, et al. Generative artificial intelligence to transform inpatient discharge summaries to patient-friendly language and format. JAMA Netw Open. 2024;7(3):e240357.
28. Achiam J, et al. Gpt-4 technical report. arXiv. 2023. Preprint arXiv:2303.08774.
29. Lyu Q, et al. Translating radiology reports into plain language using ChatGPT and GPT-4 with prompt learning: results, limitations, and potential. Visual Comput Industry Biomed Art. 2023;6(1):9.
30. Jeblick K, et al. ChatGPT makes medicine easy to swallow: an exploratory case study on simplified radiology reports. Eur Radiol. 2024;34(5):2817–25.
31. Joseph S, et al. Multilingual simplification of medical texts. arXiv. 2023. Preprint arXiv:2305.12532.
32. Tepe M, Emekli E. Decoding medical jargon: the use of AI language models (ChatGPT-4, BARD, microsoft copilot) in radiology reports. Patient Educ Couns. 2024;126:108307.
33. Apathy NC, et al. Documentation dynamics: note composition, burden, and physician efficiency. Health Serv Res. 2023;58(3):674–85.
34. Giorgi J, et al. Wanglab at mediqa-chat 2023: clinical note generation from doctor-patient conversations using large language models. arXiv. 2023. Preprint arXiv:2305.02220.
35. Biswas A, Talukdar W. Intelligent clinical documentation: harnessing generative AI for patient-centric clinical note generation. arXiv. 2024. Preprint arXiv:2405.18346.
36. Radford A, et al. Robust speech recognition via large-scale weak supervision. In: International conference on machine learning. PMLR; 2023.
37. Michalopoulos G, et al. MedicalSum: a guided clinical abstractive summarization model for generating medical reports from patient-doctor conversations. In: Findings of the Association for Computational Linguistics: EMNLP 2022; 2022.
38. Decker H, et al. Large language model– based chatbot vs surgeon-generated informed consent documentation for common procedures. JAMA Netw Open. 2023;6(10):e2336997.
39. Yang B, et al. Customizing general-purpose foundation models for medical report generation. arXiv. 2023. Preprint arXiv:2306.05642.
40. Be the provider of the future. [cited 13 August 2024]; Available from: https://regard.com/.
41. Gliadkovskaya A. Banner Health rolls out Regard's AI tool to streamline diagnoses, clinical documentation. 2024 [cited 20 August 2024]; Available from: https://www.fiercehealthcare.com/providers/banner-health-rolls-out-regard-tool-streamline-clinical-documentation.

42. Introducing Microsoft 365 Copilot — your copilot for work. [cited 20 August 2024]; Available from: https://news.microsoft.com/reinventing-productivity/.
43. Team G, et al. Gemini: a family of highly capable multimodal models. arXiv. 2023. Preprint arXiv:2312.11805.
44. Zhang P, Kamel Boulos MN. Generative AI in medicine and healthcare: promises, opportunities and challenges. Future Internet. 2023;15(9):286.
45. Nova K. Generative AI in healthcare: advancements in electronic health records, facilitating medical languages, and personalized patient care. J Adv Anal Healthcare Manag. 2023;7(1):115–31.
46. Reddy S. Generative AI in healthcare: an implementation science informed translational path on application, integration and governance. Implement Sci. 2024;19(1):27.
47. Clough RAJ, et al. Transforming healthcare documentation: harnessing the potential of AI to generate discharge summaries. BJGP Open. 2024;8(1).
48. Hartman VC, et al. A method to automate the discharge summary hospital course for neurology patients. J Am Med Inform Assoc. 2023;30(12):1995–2003.
49. Van Veen D, et al. Adapted large language models can outperform medical experts in clinical text summarization. Nat Med. 2024;30(4):1134–42.
50. Wang J, et al. PhenoPad: building AI enabled note-taking interfaces for patient encounters. NPJ Digit Med. 2022;5(1):12.
51. Adedeji A, Joshi S, Doohan B. The sound of healthcare: improving medical transcription ASR accuracy with large language models. arXiv. 2024. Preprint arXiv:2402.07658.
52. Northwestern Medicine deploys DAX Copilot embedded in Epic within its enterprise to improve patient and physician experiences. 2024 [cited 20 August 2024]; Available from: https://news.nuance.com/2024-08-15-Northwestern-Medicine-deploys-DAX-Copilot-embedded-in-Epic-within-its-enterprise-to-improve-patient-and-physician-experiences.
53. Providence and Microsoft enable AI innovation at scale to improve the future of care. 2024 [cited 20 August 2024]; Available from: https://news.nuance.com/2024-03-08-Providence-and-Microsoft-Enable-AI-Innovation-at-Scale-to-Improve-the-Future-of-Care.
54. WellSpan health advances its leadership in delivering exceptional provider and patient experience with Nuance DAX Copilot. [cited 20 August 2024]; Available from: https://news.nuance.com/2024-03-07-WellSpan-Health-Advances-Its-Leadership-in-Delivering-Exceptional-Provider-and-Patient-Experience-with-Nuance-DAX-Copilot.
55. Intermountain health Deploys DAX Copilot across the enterprise to empower clinicians and administrators with data-driven insights to transform healthcare delivery, costs and outcomes. [cited 20 August 2024]; Available from: https://news.nuance.com/2024-05-02-Intermountain-Health-Deploys-DAX-Copilot-Across-the-Enterprise-to-Empower-Clinicians-and-Administrators-With-Data-Driven-Insights-to-Transform-Healthcare-Delivery-Costs-and-Outcomes.
56. Suki, enterprise-grade AI assistant. [cited 13 August 2024]; Available from: https://www.suki.ai/suki-assistant/.
57. Beavins E. Suki brings AI scribes to community health centers with limited cash flow. 2024 [cited 20 August 2024]; Available from: https://www.fiercehealthcare.com/ai-and-machine-learning/suki-brings-ai-scribes-community-health-centers-limited-cash-flow.
58. Garcia P, et al. Artificial intelligence–generated draft replies to patient inbox messages. JAMA Netw Open. 2024;7(3):e243201.
59. Ellen AI-Your smart AI companion with voice. [cited 13 August 2024]; Available from: https://round-spear-8489.typedream.app/.
60. Yang X, et al. Gatortron: a large clinical language model to unlock patient information from unstructured electronic health records. arXiv. 2022. Preprint arXiv:2203.03540.
61. Peng C, et al. A study of generative large language model for medical research and healthcare. NPJ Digit Med. 2023;6(1):210.
62. Zakka C, et al. Almanac Copilot: towards autonomous electronic health record navigation. arXiv. 2024. Preprint arXiv:2405.07896.

63. Harrison JE, et al. ICD-11: an international classification of diseases for the twenty-first century. BMC Med Inform Decis Mak. 2021;21:1–10.
64. World Health Organization. International classification of diseases 11th revision. 2024 [cited 13 August 2024]; Available from: https://icd.who.int/en.
65. Toner E, et al. Financial impact of inaccurate coding plus cost-effectiveness analysis for surgically managed patients with periprosthetic fractures. Cureus. 2021;13(2).
66. Yang Z, et al. Surpassing GPT-4 medical coding with a two-stage approach. arXiv. 2023. Preprint arXiv:2311.13735.
67. Li R, Wang X, Yu H, Exploring LLM multi-agents for ICD coding. arXiv. 2024. Preprint arXiv:2406.15363.
68. Corti code-AI-powered medical coding. [cited 13 August 2024]; Available from: https://www.corti.ai/solutions/code.
69. Tung JYM, et al. Comparison of the quality of discharge letters written by large language models and junior clinicians: single-blinded study. J Med Internet Res. 2024;26:e57721.
70. Yakovchuk O, Vasin M. Increasing the accuracy of handwriting text recognition in medical prescriptions with generative artificial intelligence. Technol Audit Prod Reserv. 2023;4(2/72):18–21.
71. Sai S, et al. Generative ai for transformative healthcare: a comprehensive study of emerging models, applications, case studies and limitations. IEEE Access. 2024;2:231–235.
72. Neelima BD, et al. Generative AI–the revolutionizing virtual agents in health care. Int Res J Adv Eng Hub (IRJAEH). 2024;2(02):231–5.
73. Jiang LY, et al. Health system-scale language models are all-purpose prediction engines. Nature. 2023;619(7969):357–62.
74. Lataran PN, et al. Developing a BERT-enhanced blockchain model for HealthInsurance fraud detection. J Inform Syst Res Pract. 2024;2(3):56–61.
75. Choudhury A, Shamszare H. Investigating the impact of user trust on the adoption and use of ChatGPT: survey analysis. J Med Internet Res. 2023;25:e47184.
76. Ji Z, et al. Survey of hallucination in natural language generation. ACM Comput Surv. 2023;55(12):1–38.
77. Fui-Hoon Nah F, et al. Generative AI and ChatGPT: applications, challenges, and AI-human collaboration. Taylor & Francis; 2023. p. 277–304.
78. Salazar GZ, et al. Efficacy of AI Chats to determine an emergency: a comparison between OpenAI's ChatGPT, Google Bard, and Microsoft Bing AI Chat. Cureus. 2023;15(9).
79. Ji S, et al. A unified review of deep learning for automated medical coding. ACM Comput Surv. 2022;25:14–25.
80. Tustumi F, Andreollo NA, Aguilar-Nascimento JEd. Future of the language models in healthcare: the role of chatGPT. ABCD. arquivos brasileiros de cirurgia digestiva (são paulo). 2023;36:e1727.
81. Varghese J, Chapiro J. ChatGPT: the transformative influence of generative AI on science and healthcare. J Hepatol. 2024;80(6):977–80.
82. Wang C, et al. Ethical considerations of using ChatGPT in health care. J Med Internet Res. 2023;25:e48009.
83. Clement T, et al. Xair: a systematic metareview of explainable ai (xai) aligned to the software development process. Mach Learn Knowl Extract. 2023;5(1):78–108.
84. Balloccu S, et al. Leak, cheat, repeat: data contamination and evaluation malpractices in closed-source llms. arXiv. 2024. Preprint arXiv:2402.03927.
85. Chen H, et al. Knowledge distillation for closed-source language models. arXiv. 2024. Preprint arXiv:2401.07013.

Application of Generative AI in Patient Engagement

Mohammad ZareiNejad and Parisa Tavana

1 Introduction

Artificial Intelligence (AI) applications in healthcare are still in their early stages [1]. Robotic surgery [2], electronic health records [3], remote patient monitoring devices [4], predictive analytics tools [5], telemedicine [6], and virtual health assistants [7] are just a few ways AI technology is being used in the healthcare sector to enhance patient outcomes and patient-centered care solutions [1]. It should be noted that today, access to information has increased with technological advancements, making patients more aware of their conditions and care options than ever before [8]. Reducing risks and improving patient health outcomes are current challenges faced by healthcare systems worldwide [9]. Engaging the active voice of patients is becoming a prominent ideology in healthcare, with significant implications for patient experiences, health outcomes, and healthcare research and funding [10]. Engagement with treatment support tools is directly associated with improved reliability, recovery, and more consistent attendance at treatment sessions while reducing dropout rates [11].

M. ZareiNejad
Department of Computer Engineering, South Tehran Branch, Islamic Azad University, Tehran, Iran
e-mail: St_m_zareinejad@azad.ac.ir

P. Tavana (✉)
Department of Computer Engineering, Science and Research Branch, Islamic Azad University, Tehran, Iran
e-mail: parisa.tavana@srbiau.ac.ir

A. Zamanifar, M. Faezipour (eds.), *Application of Generative AI in Healthcare Systems*, https://doi.org/10.1007/978-3-031-82963-5_5

1.1 The Role and Definitions of Patient Engagement

Patient engagement is considered a precursor to quality, patient-centered care that ultimately contributes to improving care quality [12]. Engaging patients in responsibly managing their health is widely recognized as a way to address these challenges. In fact, it has been shown that patients who actively and effectively manage their healthcare achieve more positive clinical outcomes compared to those who are passive or less engaged [13]. Real-time monitoring, predictive analytics, and iterative improvements ensure that this strategy enhances efficiency and cost-effectiveness within the healthcare ecosystem [1]. Additionally, there is growing consensus that patient engagement is a crucial factor for improving the quality of care and increasing patient safety [14]. Patients are defined as one of the key stakeholders in healthcare and decision-making, underscoring the necessity of their involvement in the treatment process [15]. The rising interest in patient engagement is occurring at a time when healthcare costs in Canada are steadily increasing—in 2016, healthcare costs were estimated to reach $228 billion, comprising 11% of Canada's GDP [16]. Ensuring the sustainability and growth of healthcare services in Canada has thus become a top priority [16]. It has also been suggested that declining trust in the Canadian healthcare system requires increased public engagement to drive critical reforms in this area [17]. Study [13] states that to fully understand patient engagement and introduce some terms, it is helpful to distinguish this concept from others used in the literature to describe aspects of the process by which patients become actively involved in their healthcare. Indeed, studies discussing the active role of patients often use various terms (i.e., patient engagement, patient activation, patient involvement, patient participation, patient adherence/compliance, and patient empowerment) interchangeably [18]. Each term has its specific meaning related to the role patients play in engaging with their healthcare [13].

A recent component of the ongoing commitment to patient engagement is the increased interest and investment specifically in patient engagement in health research [19]. This concept of engagement goes beyond viewing patients merely as subjects or participants in research; it reflects the increasing demand for more ethical, democratic, and moral healthcare practices [19]. Study [19] states that the paradigm shift towards patient engagement in health research provides opportunities for greater impact on the three central goals of patient-centered care. This shift requires researchers, clinicians, and healthcare administrators to view patients as active and respected partners in the research process. Indeed, as the ultimate recipients of health research findings, patients are the most important stakeholders. As a result, this scenario represents an ideal in healthcare, where patients are well-informed and motivated to engage in their own medical care. This is a way to ensure that patients receive care that is appropriate to their characteristics, needs, preferences, and individual conditions [20].

The definition of patient engagement according to the study [21], is as follows: "A set of behaviors by patients, family members, and healthcare professionals, as well as a set of organizational policies and practices that involve patients and family members as active members of the healthcare team and collaborative partnerships with providers and healthcare delivery organizations, with the desirable goals of improving the quality and safety of healthcare." This definition views engagement as a systemic concept that results from patient actions across different levels of complexity (i.e., individual, relational, organizational, and health policy levels) [13]. In another study [22], the dynamic and multi-dimensional nature of patient engagement is described, defining it as "a multi-dimensional psychosocial process resulting from the simultaneous enactment of cognitive, emotional, and behavioral aspects by individuals regarding their health status and its management." These authors specifically highlight the role of emotional processing, alongside cognitive and behavioral activation, as a critical component in the process of fully engaging patients in their healthcare [13]. Figure 1 illustrates the patient engagement process.

Despite these differences in definitions, the literature in this field generally supports the notion that the term "patient" should not be limited to someone who merely receives care [19]. It refers to any individual or group with lived experience related to a health issue or healthcare system, including family members, caregivers, and organizations involved with the targeted population [23]. Based on all these definitions, the study [13] states that patient engagement is a complex and multifaceted experience that cannot be reduced merely to the patient's ability to adhere to medical prescriptions. Specifically, patient engagement is characterized by the following aspects:

- *Behavioral aspect (what the patient does)*: This relates to all the activities a patient undertakes to cope with illness and treatments [13].

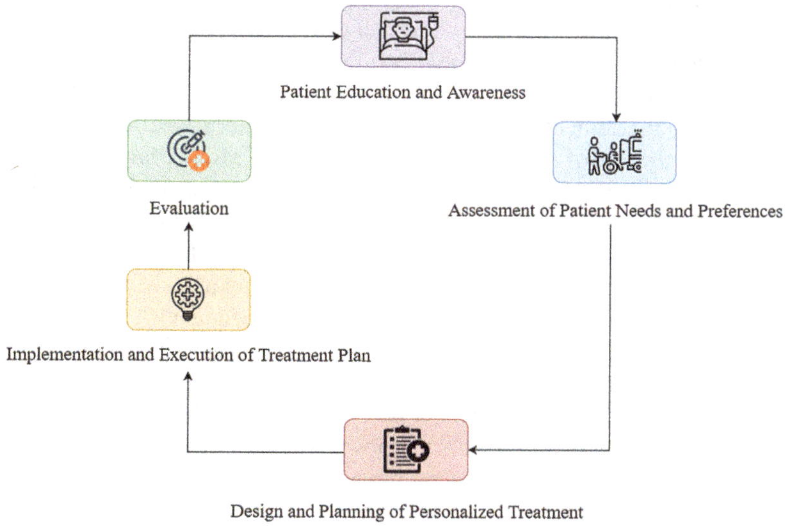

Fig. 1 Streamlining patient engagement

- *Cognitive aspect (what the patient thinks and knows)*: This pertains to the patient's knowledge and understanding of the illness, treatments, potential progress, and monitoring of the disease [13].
- *Emotional aspect (what the patient feels)*: This involves the psychological and emotional reactions a patient experiences while adapting to the onset of illness and the new life conditions associated with it [13].

Over the past 10 years, patient engagement in health research has emerged as a new phase in healthcare delivery; it offers an opportunity to involve patients in decision-making related to health research while improving health outcomes [24]. There are several reasons for advancing patient engagement in health research, which are grounded in ethical, outcome-driven, and moral value systems [25]. Despite these overarching values, there is limited agreement on how to involve patients throughout the research process, stemming from a limited understanding of the meaning, conceptualization, and activities of engagement, leading to hesitant adoption [26].

1.2 AI and Patient Engagement in Healthcare

In the study [27], the authors state that artificial intelligence has penetrated nearly every field in recent years, from smartphones, watches, washing machines, and more to smart homes and even smart cities. AI has been significantly used in the healthcare sector in recent years. AI can be employed in various diagnostic and treatment areas, including patient monitoring, robotic surgeries, data analysis, patient risk assessments, drug discovery, and clinical trials. AI technologies can generally be divided into machine learning, computer vision, natural language processing (NLP), deep learning, and context-aware processing, which can be combined to provide solutions for different healthcare issues. A study [28] states that one of our tasks is to understand patients' opinions regarding the use of AI in their care. Along with investments in AI, there have been numerous calls to gather public perspectives on the use of AI not only in healthcare but also in various other fields. It is important to answer these questions: How can we responsibly research patient engagement with AI, considering the criticisms and the risks and shortcomings reported in AI-supported technologies in healthcare? How should academic researchers respond responsibly to the calls from policymakers and providers to initiate new forms of patient engagement with AI advancements?

There is an urgent need to examine the role of inviting patient participation as part of the social discussion about the emergence of AI. Promising statements about an impending AI revolution are everywhere [29], and healthcare is currently the largest area of AI investment [30]. An AI-powered control center at Johns Hopkins allowed staff to assign emergency department (ED) patients to hospital beds 30% faster [27]. However, there is growing evidence of the harmful consequences of AI-supported tools in healthcare [31], such as potential misdiagnoses, incorrect treatments, and unfair disparities in care outcomes. Patient engagement is one of the important stakeholders in healthcare, creating controversial views regarding their potential involvement in various aspects of healthcare [8]. Despite the mentioned benefits, some studies have shown mixed results. Findings from a study on patient-reported outcome measures indicated that providing feedback to patients did not have a significant clinical impact on patient empowerment or satisfaction [32]. As part of mitigating these risks, recent scientific articles on machine learning and artificial intelligence highlight the importance of "patient engagement," "patient involvement," or "patient representation" in achieving responsible governance and providing effective guidance for the implementation of AI in healthcare [28]. However, it is unclear how this enthusiasm for patient engagement practices relates to the numerous skeptical and negative evaluations of such practices, as well as recent critical perspectives on (medical) AI [28]. Several researchers have turned their attention to what is known as "leftist critiques" of AI [33] including attention to "health data justice" [34]. Organizations like Google and IBM are working on integrating AI into healthcare. Most AI-based healthcare applications use Google's Deepmind Health or IBM's Watson to diagnose specific diseases after collecting data from mobile applications [35].

The study [28] states that researching patient engagement with emerging technologies, such as AI-supported medical applications, is not straightforward, as many of these developments are still in their early stages and are transitioning from data science and computer science environments to early explorations in clinical settings. Even though citizens may have little experience with direct interaction with AI-supported healthcare tools, AI is gradually affecting patient care as part of complex and distributed socio-technical healthcare systems. In these systems, AI manifests in various forms, including AI-assisted computation of patient risk profiles (prognosis) and eligibility for procedures (triage) as part of clinical decision support systems; setting medical imaging devices and diagnostic evaluation of digital scans and patient tissue slides (diagnosis); and generating medical reports using automated speech recognition and appointment scheduling software (management). In several AI policy documents, "discourse on engagement" is invoked in the context of "building trust" or "acceptance" for AI systems [36]. A study [27] indicates that the complexity of current medicines, which require a vast amount of information for analysis, is directly linked to the increased use of AI in the healthcare industry. Additionally, there are not enough researchers to meet the demand for studies. Therefore, AI applications, by leveraging advanced computation, assist researchers in hospitals to overcome the limitations of human intelligence in the medical field. Consequently, AI offers various benefits, including ease of performing complex calculations, increased accuracy, analyzing data collected from various sources, solving complex problems in less time, and making effective decisions.

Over the past decades, various forms of patient engagement, such as patient consultations, invited engagement events, patient representation in decision-making bodies, research participation, and co-design of medical methods and systems by patients, have been intertwined with concepts and meanings [28]. The World Health Organization (WHO) in the Western Pacific region closely collaborates with member countries to implement health-related programs by strengthening regulations and policies and improving oversight of patient safety practices. Among the key initiatives are the efforts of the WHO and member countries to enhance the engagement of patients, families, and communities in their own healthcare. These efforts include focusing on patient needs at the center of care, ensuring patients fully understand the proposed treatment, and obtaining informed consent from them. Additionally, pandemics and widespread outbreaks can claim millions of lives, disrupt communities, and devastate economies. In this regard, the WHO Health Emergencies Program (WHE), in collaboration with member countries, helps them prepare to respond to widespread outbreaks and pandemics [37]. Studies have shown that meaningful patient engagement can reduce the burden of harm by up to 15%, save countless lives each year, and save billions of dollars [37].

Patient engagement has been proposed as a means to enhance the efficiency, sustainability, and quality of medical innovations, increase options for individual patients, democratize decision-making in healthcare, empower patients, and promote equitable and fair medical practices [38]. On the other hand, AI is rapidly evolving in the healthcare sector, and this trend is expected to continue. The use of new technologies in this industry allows physicians to provide continuous responses, notifications, and immediate reminders. Patients benefit from reduced waiting times and faster access to care. AI-powered tools can recognize and analyze patients' faces, emotions, and behaviors to deliver personalized responses, leading to increased patient satisfaction. Personalized healthcare recommendations generated by AI tools have improved health outcomes and patient satisfaction while promoting preventive measures [1]. The capacity for AI-driven patient engagement to enhance innovative care is one of its key advantages [39]. A study [1] states that AI-based patient engagement has emerged as a transformative force in healthcare, showing that it can lead to better outcomes, increased patient empowerment, and significant cost savings. The future of healthcare holds great promise as we continue to harness the power of AI and data-driven insights with a patient-centered approach at its core. It is important to note that generative AI in patient engagement today holds significant potential to improve healthcare processes. This technology can not only be effective in diagnosing and treating diseases but also play a crucial role in increasing transparency, flexibility, and patient involvement in health decision-making. However, to optimally exploit this technology, it is necessary to address the ethical challenges and issues related to patient privacy and trust. The connection and approaches between AI and patient engagement indicate that this combination can be used as a powerful tool to improve healthcare services and patient experience in healthcare systems [1].

2 Generative Artificial Intelligence

Tom Freston is credited with the saying, "Innovation is taking two things that exist and putting them together in a new way." For a long time in history, it was commonly assumed that artistic and creative works such as writing poetry, creating software, designing fashion, and composing music were activities only humans could perform. This assumption has been drastically altered by recent advances in artificial intelligence, which can generate new content that is indistin-guishable from human skills [40]. Generative AI refers to deep learning models that can produce high-quality content based on the training data used. Simply put, a generative model applies what it has learned from training data to create entirely new content. This is why it is called "generative," meaning "producer." Studies indicate that generative AI has a wide range of applications. If you are active in the art world, you can use this technology to create new music pieces, visual art, and even new poems. In the business world, you can use it to generate realistic synthetic data for testing or training. In the medical field, generative AI is utilized to create synthetic medical images for research purposes. In any field where individuals are active, it is enough to identify the potential of your domain and use Generative AI (GenAI) to improve the quality and speed of your work processes. Figure 2 introduces some of the most widely used generative AI models in each domain.

Generative AI is used in various fields, including generating news content, writing articles, translating texts, composing music, creating images, and even producing advertising content. Due to its ability to generate large-scale content quickly and accurately, generative AI has become a powerful tool for individuals and companies, significantly reducing the time and costs associated with content production and improving content quality. Research has reported that the global market for

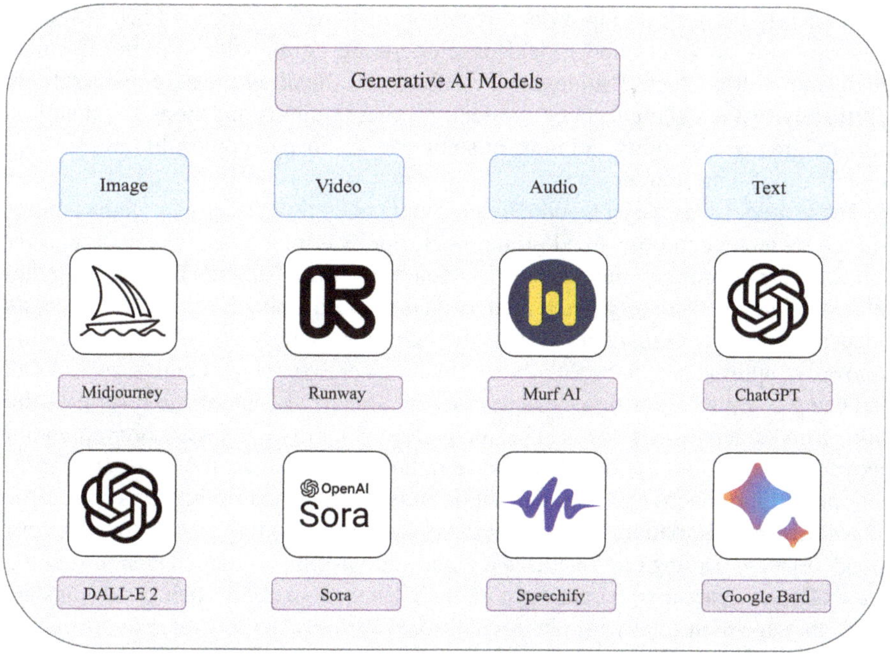

Fig. 2 Some of the most widely used generative AI models in each domain

generative AI was valued at $10.79 billion in 2022. It is predicted that this market will reach approximately $118.06 billion by 2032, with a compound annual growth rate (CAGR) of 27.02% from 2023 to 2032 [41]. These effects are remarkable not only for the community of information science and business systems, where we will face revolutionary opportunities but also for the challenges and risks that we must address and manage to steer the technology and its responsible and sustainable use toward a desirable and sustainable direction [40]. Additionally, the increasing access to large-scale data sets, along with advances in deep learning techniques, has driven the rapid development of generative AI [41]. By leveraging generative AI capabilities in healthcare, providers can empower patients to participate in their care and foster a collaborative and personalized approach to healthcare delivery [43]. In essence, generative AI acts as a catalyst for patient empowerment, transcending traditional healthcare paradigms and ushering in a new era of personalized and patient-centered care [43].

However, amid the excitement and promise of generative AI in healthcare, it is crucial to examine the ethical considerations and challenges associated with its adoption. Questions about data privacy, algorithmic bias, and the ethical implications of AI-based decision-making are numerous and require thoughtful reflection and responsible implementation [42]. Despite its impressive potential, generative AI also has limitations. These AI models require large amounts of data and computational resources for training and may inadvertently produce inappropriate content. Therefore, their final performance requires careful attention and oversight. It is important to note that bias, racism, deception, and sensationalist propaganda may inadvertently be used as input data, resulting in flawed outcomes [43]. However, generative AI providers and model developers are continually working on these models to address such challenges and adhere to ethical and legal considerations. Ultimately, as GenAI creates new content, it raises complex questions about authorship and ownership rights and may, in some cases, infringe copyright laws through the misuse of data sources.

These models can assist healthcare providers in creating treatment plans tailored to each patient's conditions and preferences. For example, AI can generate optimal solutions for improving interactions between doctors and patients by analyzing data related to medical history, treatment behaviors, and patients' personal interests. Focusing on patient engagement with the help of generative AI is one of the most innovative approaches in the healthcare field. Generative AI, leveraging patient data and using complex algorithms, can produce personalized content and responses that align with each patient's needs. This technology not only enhances communication between patients and the healthcare system but also promotes more effective interactions and more active patient participation in the treatment process. Applications of generative AI in patient engagement may include providing personalized recommendations, managing chronic diseases, and supporting treatment decision-making. For example, generative AI can help patients learn more about their conditions and better manage their treatment plans. Additionally, this technology can assist doctors in updating their treatment plans based on new data. Generative AI can play a role in creating more accurate patient profiles, enabling healthcare providers to design more personalized treatment plans. By analyzing both historical and real-time data, these systems can gain a better understanding of patients' behaviors and treatment patterns. Such an approach leads to trust-based interactions and increased patient satisfaction. Moreover, one of the main advantages of using generative AI in patient engagement is the improvement in patients' quality of life. With this technology, patients can access more accurate information and take an active role in their treatment decision-making. This not only helps improve treatment outcomes but also increases patient satisfaction with the treatment process. Additionally, generative AI can act as an intelligent intermediary, translating complex medical information into simple and understandable language for patients. This process helps improve patients' understanding of their health status and prepares them for active participation in treatment decision-making. This technology can also foster more dynamic and reciprocal interactions in the treatment process by providing real-time, patient-specific treatment recommendations.

As a result, the use of generative AI in patient engagement can lead to significant improvements in the quality of healthcare services. However, to optimize the use of this technology, further research and attention to existing challenges are necessary. Improving data security techniques, increasing the accuracy of generative models, and establishing appropriate legal frameworks can accelerate the adoption and widespread use of generative AI in this field. In summary, generative AI can contribute to creating a more dynamic and collaborative treatment environment, where patients are not only recipients of care but also active partners in the treatment process. This chapter will explore the different types of generative AI models that have gained popularity in patient engagement, followed by an examination of the applications and challenges in this field.

2.1 Generative Adversarial Networks

Ian Goodfellow introduced Generative Adversarial Networks (GANs) in 2014. This deep learning technique presented a new approach to organizing competing neural networks for generating and then ranking content variations, which can realistically produce people, voices, music, and text. This work inspired the exploration of how generative AI could be used to create realistic deepfakes that mimic voices and individuals in videos. GANs are a novel class of deep generative models that have recently garnered significant attention [44]. These networks learn by extracting backpropagation signals through a competitive process involving a pair of networks [45]. The study [46] states that since the discovery of neural networks, there has been a trend toward training data (structured or unstructured) and predicting outcomes based on these training sets. However, new neural networks, particularly GANs, are gaining popularity due to their ability to generate new data rather than classify it. GANs emerged as an advanced framework in deep learning, revolutionizing the generation of artificial data by placing two neurons against each other in a competitive learning algorithm. GANs have proven to be a powerful tool for the automated processing of information in fields such as computer vision, natural language processing, healthcare, and design generation [47].

GANs have achieved remarkable results in various image synthesis tasks and have become a prominent topic in computer vision research due to their significant performance across diverse applications [48]. GANs use two neural networks that operate against each other and can be trained simultaneously through simple feedback. Their adaptive learning capabilities enable the generation of new data without replicating previous results. Figure 3 shows how a basic GAN model works. Due to these advantages, GANs have found widespread applications in the medical and healthcare sectors. Fundamental applications such as image segmentation, image-to-image translation, style transfer, and classification have become increasingly recognized. The study [49] states that Artificial Intelligence has been introduced as one of the key technological innovations of the twenty-first century. In healthcare, significant attention is focused on the ability of AI inference systems to analyze large datasets to find patterns that would be impossible to program. Generative AI, including generative adversarial networks, is a new type of machine learning that works to create fake data after learning the features of real data. Artificially generated synthetic data has the potential to transform clinical research and protect patient privacy. Using innovative techniques, it is increasingly possible to completely anonymize datasets so that no data can be traced back to a real individual. This can be used to expand and balance datasets as well as replace the use of real patient data in some cases. In the dynamic and growing landscape of healthcare, generative AI has emerged as a transformative and novel technology with multifaceted benefits. This technology helps patients become more involved in their treatment processes and allows doctors to tailor treatment plans to the individual characteristics of patients. Generative AI can help enhance patient engagement by creating intelligent question-and-answer systems [50], providing medical advice, and developing customized treatment plans [51]. The following section introduces and examines GAN-based models used in patient engagement.

Engagement is typically measured through patient reports, which may be prone to response bias. Additionally, the variable use of different questionnaires makes it

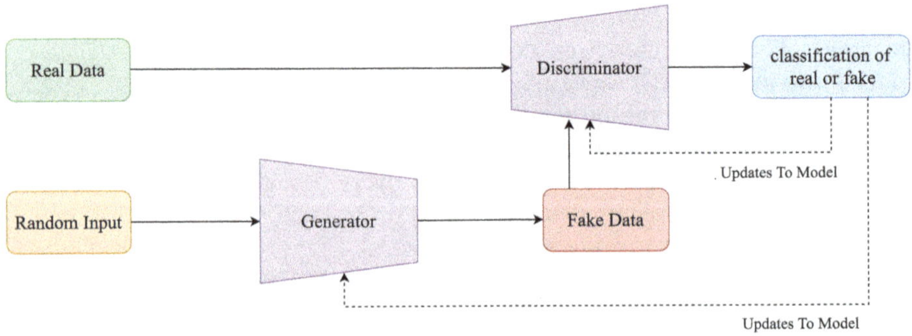

Fig. 3 How a basic GAN model works

challenging to compare patient engagement across different health systems [52]. In the study [52], the authors investigate the MET (Multimodal Perception of Engagement for Telehealth) algorithm, designed to evaluate the level of patient engagement in remote therapy sessions. Currently, providers are implementing telehealth services without clear guidance on how to improve or measure patient engagement remotely. For example, the sudden shift to virtual care to prevent the transmission of COVID-19 did not allow providers to receive training on using technology-based care beyond initial orientation to web-based platforms. This algorithm is implemented in a semi-supervised GAN (generative adversarial network) framework based on emotional and cognitive features that are widely used in the psychology literature, utilizing latent vectors. The authors aim to better understand patient engagement in remote therapy sessions in the mental health domain. Additionally, in this study, the authors released the MEDICA dataset, which includes 1299 video clips, each 3 s long, and conducted tests to evaluate the quality of their approach. These videos are labeled with eight emotions related to mental health: happiness, sadness, anger, neutrality, anxiety, embarrassment, fear, and surprise. MEDICA was created by collecting mock therapy session videos made publicly available by various medical psychiatry faculties for training their students. The proposed framework reports a 40% improvement in root mean square error (RMSE) over existing advanced methods in engagement estimation. In real-world experiments, it was also observed that there are positive correlations between scores on the working alliance questionnaire reported by psychotherapists. These results indicate the potential of the proposed model in providing patient engagement estimates that align with the engagement metrics used by psychotherapists [52].

2.1.1 GANs for Synthetic EHR Data and Privacy Protection

GANs play a transformative role in patient engagement by generating synthetic Electronic Health Record (EHR) data. These synthetic datasets can mimic real patient data without compromising individual privacy, a crucial element in healthcare research and development. Using GANs for synthetic EHR generation ensures that sensitive patient information remains confidential, yet still allows for large-scale data analysis and algorithm training. By doing so, patient trust is maintained, and researchers can explore new ways of improving patient engagement, care delivery, and personalized treatments without risking data breaches. This aligns with patient engagement efforts by allowing safer, more robust machine learning models to be trained on diverse, representative data while minimizing risks. In today's healthcare landscape, there is an increasing emphasis on empowering patients to actively participate in their health journeys, with the core of this paradigm shift being the integration of generative artificial intelligence (AI) technologies, which have tremendous potential to transform the patient experience [42]. A study [53] states that access to electronic health record (EHR) data has provided an impetus for computational advances in medical research. Sharing synthetic EHR data while maintaining privacy can facilitate further research into improving the quality of care and patient experience, thereby enhancing patient engagement. However, various concerns, especially regarding privacy, can limit access to and the shared use of EHR data. Sharing synthetic EHR data can mitigate the risk. In this study, the authors propose a novel method called the medical generative adversarial network (medGAN) to generate synthetic records of real patients. Med-GAN can generate high-dimensional discrete variables (such as binary features and counts) from real patient record inputs using a combination of an autoencoder and generative adversarial networks. To demonstrate feasibility, med-GAN has been shown to produce synthetic patient records that perform comparably to real data in various tests, including distribution statistics, predictive modeling tasks, and evaluations by medical experts.

2.1.2 GAN-Powered SeqMed for Drug Combination Prediction

In the realm of patient engagement, GANs can assist in drug combination predictions, providing a personalized approach to healthcare. By analyzing complex datasets, GANs can generate novel drug combinations that may be more effective for specific patient profiles. This application not only improves treatment outcomes but also enhances patient involvement in their care. With more accurate predictions of potential side effects and efficacy, patients can be empowered to make informed decisions about their treatment options. Moreover, these models can dramatically reduce the time required for new drug combination approvals, improving patient access to life-saving treatments and enhancing overall engagement with healthcare providers. In study [54], the authors propose the SeqMed model, a sequential generative model for predicting drug combinations. Leveraging the power of Generative Adversarial Nets, SeqMed is able to obtain a descriptive representation of a patient's medical records and provide precise drug recommendations for that patient. Experiments on real electronic medical record (EMR) datasets, MIMIC-III, show that SeqMed significantly outperforms previous methods and can consistently converge. The results obtained from the SeqMed model indicate a 5.81% and 6.49% improvement in Jaccard and f1-score metrics, respectively, compared to recent advanced methods for predicting drug combinations. These advancements can contribute to improving the accuracy of drug recommendations and, consequently, enhancing the quality of treatment management in patients with complex conditions.

2.1.3 GANs in Predictive Healthcare

GANs are increasingly being employed in predictive healthcare, where they assist in forecasting disease progression, treatment outcomes, and even patient behavior. Their ability to generate realistic datasets allows healthcare providers to anticipate patient needs more accurately, fostering a proactive approach to care. For example, GANs can predict hospital readmission risks or help in preventive healthcare by analyzing lifestyle data alongside medical records. This enhances patient engagement as individuals can be informed earlier about potential health risks and receive tailored interventions before complications arise. Ultimately, this improves communication between patients and healthcare providers, aligning well with a more patient-centric healthcare model. GenAI can predict future health trends based on current patient data. These predictions help patients proactively participate in managing their health. For example, by analyzing a patient's health data, GenAI might identify an increased risk of heart disease, which could encourage the patient to make lifestyle changes, such as adopting a healthier diet and engaging in regular exercise, to prevent or delay the onset of the disease. For instance, in study [55], the authors demonstrate the importance of using real-world heart attack datasets to validate research findings. In this context, thorough reviews have shown that the CTGAN model (a synthetic data generation model) has significantly outperformed expectations in generating synthetic heart attack data. Additionally, in the classification phase, the TabNet architecture has outperformed all previous deep learning and machine learning methods. This study highlights the capabilities of deep generative models in producing high-quality synthetic data for heart attack research. The research results indicate that using interpretable TabNet models offers superior performance in heart attack classification compared to traditional machine learning methods. These advancements suggest that integrating advanced technologies such as AI and deep generative models can effectively improve the diagnosis and prediction of heart attacks, which in turn can lead to increased survival rates and better health management for patients.

2.1.4 GANs for Cardiovascular Disease Prediction and Risk Assessment

Cardiovascular diseases (CVD) are among the leading causes of death globally, making early detection and risk assessment crucial. GANs can be employed to predict the likelihood of CVD by generating synthetic yet accurate patient data based on various risk factors like genetics, lifestyle, and pre-existing conditions. These models allow healthcare professionals to better identify at-risk individuals, thus enabling earlier interventions. From a patient engagement perspective, this proactive approach allows patients to take an active role in managing their cardiovascular health. They can be given personalized recommendations and resources, making the healthcare experience more collaborative and empowering. In a similar study [56], generative adversarial networks were used to improve risk assessment. For this research, data from 1700 individuals, including carotid ultrasound results and coronary angiography scores (CAS), the gold standard for determining the extent of coronary artery stenosis, were examined. In these data, 52 different factors were considered and divided into three subgroups: (i) factors related to office examinations, (ii) laboratory-related factors, and (iii) carotid ultrasonic imaging features. To address the imbalance in risk groups, the "Synthetic Minority Over-sampling Technique" (SMOTE) was used. The performance of the GAN model was evaluated using five-fold cross-validation and compared with LSTM and RNN models. The results showed that the GAN model achieved an accuracy of 93.00% and an AUC score of 0.953, outperforming the LSTM and RNN models, which achieved accuracies of 85.80% and 82.50%, with AUC scores of 0.920 and 0.881, respectively.

2.2 *Large Language Models*

Artificial intelligence, as an interdisciplinary science, has always been striving to develop methods and algorithms that enable computers to process and understand natural human language. One of the significant advancements in this field is the emergence of large language models, which have improved text analysis capabilities. Large language models (LLMs) are a type of advanced machine model in the field of natural language processing. These models, with a large number of parameters and training on a massive dataset, can intelligently generate content and respond to new texts. Recently, large language models have generated considerable interest in various domains [57]. In just a few years, large language models have gone from non-existent to ubiquitous in the discourse of machine learning [58]. A study [59] states that language is essentially a complex and challenging system of human expressions governed by grammatical rules. Developing AI algorithms capable of understanding and comprehending a language is a significant challenge. As a primary approach, language modeling has been extensively studied for language understanding and generation over the past two decades, evolving from statistical language models to neural language models [59]. Due to their unprecedented performance in various applications, large language models are gaining increasing popularity in academia and industry [60]. Figure 4 highlights the milestones in this field over recent years. Additionally, given their excellent performance in managing various applications such as general natural language tasks and domain-specific issues, LLMs are increasingly used by individuals with critical information needs, such as students or patients [60]. Large language models such as BERT [61], GPT-3 [62], GPT-4 [63], and LLaMA-2 [64], have demonstrated impressive performance in a wide range of healthcare-related tasks. They can respond to open-ended questions without being specifically trained on the task at hand, creating excitement and concern about their use in healthcare settings [65]. Many applications of LLMs have been proposed in the medical domain [58], including answering medical questions

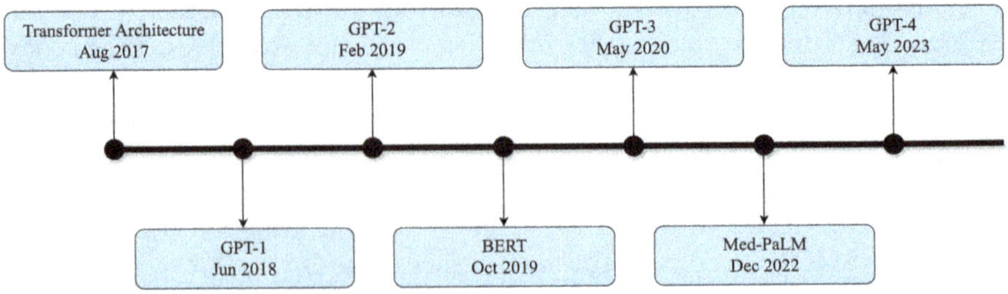

Fig. 4 Milestones of large language models over recent years

[66], extracting clinical information [67] and triage [68]. LLM chatbots are currently deployed in a wide range of biomedical fields, with impressive but varied results [65]. Recently, research on LLMs has significantly advanced in academia and industry, with a notable milestone being the launch of ChatGPT, which has attracted widespread community attention [59]. Study [69] proposes a framework for zero-shot classification of medical images using vision-language models like CLIP and LLMs like ChatGPT. The main idea is to use ChatGPT to automatically generate detailed textual descriptions of disease symptoms and visual features beyond the disease name. To address potential inaccuracies of ChatGPT on medical topics, the authors design prompts to obtain high-quality textual descriptions of identifiable visual symptoms for each disease class [70].

Rapid advancements in large language models have opened new opportunities to transform patient engagement in healthcare through conversational AI [71]. A study [71] suggests that LLMs can be used to generate customized visual cues that address an individual's background, interests, or cognitive abilities, which may improve the accuracy and specificity of tests. Similarly, multimodal LLMs can create interactive visual aids to support educational materials for patients, medical instructions, and treatment adherence reminders, making the information more engaging and comprehensible.

2.2.1 LLMs in Supporting Elderly Cognitive Health

In a study [72], LLMs were used to examine language patterns in discussions related to mental health on Reddit.[1] By analyzing 2.9 million posts in 30 subreddits from October to December 2022 and the same period in 2010, the study aimed to identify themes that align with known risk factors for suicidal thoughts [71]. The authors used Python for data processing. Empty entries or those containing only a "?" were not considered. The authors analyzed 16 subreddits related to mental health and 14 subreddits unrelated to mental health to act as controls. The study used the ConversationChain module and ConversationBufferMemory to facilitate interactive, memory-aware conversations with GPT-4. This setup enabled users to repeatedly query the model with their requests and data, ensuring a rich and coherent textual analysis of subreddit posts. By using sophisticated AI methods to interpret the nuanced language used in mental health forums, this study demonstrates how conversational AI can be useful in identifying and understanding mental health issues through user-generated content. Thus, it facilitates real-time monitoring and support and enhances the responsiveness of digital health interventions [72]. The results of this study showed that, consistent with existing theories on suicide, users in the "SuicideWatch" community primarily wrote about feelings of disconnecttion, feeling like a burden to others, hopelessness, despair, surrender, and emotional trauma. Additionally, various linguistic dimensions such as well-being,

[1] www.reddit.com

support-seeking, and distress intensity were identified across all mental health subgroups. Many of the obtained subgroup clusters aligned with the statistically based diagnostic classification system, i.e., the Hierarchical Taxonomy of Psychopathology (HiTOP), and matched the proposed categori-zations of this system. Overall, the findings of this study provide data-driven support for several language-based suicide theories and dimensional classification systems for mental health disorders. Ultimately, this new combination of natural language processing techniques can help researchers gain deeper insights into the sentiments and experiences shared on the web and may help validate or refute various mental health theories. It should be noted that this proposed approach has several limitations: the data only cover a three-month period, which may not reflect long-term patterns or seasonal variations [71]. The study is limited to Reddit and may not be generalizable to other social media platforms or offline conversations [71].

LLMs are playing an important role in supporting cognitive health among the elderly. They can assist in developing conversational agents that engage older adults in stimulating, interactive dialogues, which can help maintain cognitive function over time. Additionally, LLMs can be used in tools that offer cognitive assessments, memory training exercises, and customized content aimed at slowing cognitive decline. The ability of LLMs to adapt responses to individual users allows for highly personalized interactions, making elderly patients feel more engaged and motivated in their own cognitive health journey. Such applications align with patient engagement by encouraging active participation in cognitive exercises and fostering a sense of connection, especially for those who may experience loneliness or isolation. In another study [73], the authors utilize LLMs to prevent cognitive decline in the elderly. This study will follow two groups over the age of 70 in assisted living facilities—a control arm and a group encouraged to read books. The chatbot engages participants in the reading group by initiating conversations about the books to promote continued collaborative reading, with the hypothesis that this will measurably improve cognitive function. The chatbot is designed to make the reading experience more engaging, enjoyable, and rewarding for the participants in the intervention group. The ability of the chatbot to tailor its conversational style, content recommendations, and discussion prompts to each user's unique preferences and needs is expected to increase motivation, engagement, and adherence to the reading intervention throughout the study period. While chatbot technology has the potential to promote reading habits across various age groups, its specific aim in this study is to create a controlled environment to accurately examine the effects of increased reading on cognitive health in the elderly population. Using an AI-based assistant not only makes this type of study design possible but also opens new possibilities for personalized and scalable interventions to support healthy aging.

Generative AI tools can enhance diagnostic accuracy and clinical performance, provide quick access to precise medical information and care, and reduce workload in healthcare [74]. A study [74] states that generative AI can improve the accuracy and efficiency of treatment, communication, and outcomes with patients, support clinical decision-making, diagnostic processes, computer-aided diagnosis, and medical imaging analysis. The findings and analyses indicate that ChatGPT and machine learning-based expertise and judgment in personalized care can provide adequate treatment recommendations in accordance with the patient's clinical manifestations, disease severity, and comorbid diagnoses. ChatGPT can suggest potential diagnoses and treatment options by analyzing patient symptoms, medical history, and laboratory results. The authors discuss how improving clinical reasoning, medical education, and guideline-based healthcare management, ChatGPT can sufficiently manage medical information and provide appropriate responses to detailed questions. The study's results show that generative AI algorithms can be used in relation to clinical imaging analysis, human infection management and diagnosis, public health monitoring, patient satisfaction review, clinical infection performance and decision support systems, and microbiome-based treatments. In another study [75], the authors state that unlike traditional AI models, which often rely on structured data and predefined algorithms, LLMs excel at interpreting unstructured textual data. This feature makes them particularly useful for tasks such as real-time data interpretation, enhancing clinical decision-making, and increasing patient engagement in clinical settings. For example, LLMs can effectively screen electronic health records (EHRs) to identify important patient histories and assist physicians in interpreting complex diagnostic data.

2.2.2 LLMs for Psychotherapy and Motivational Interviewing

LLMs, like GPT models, are being applied in psychotherapy and motivational interviewing to provide scalable, conversational mental health support. These models can engage patients in therapeutic dialogues, simulate human-like conversations, and offer supportive responses, helping patients navigate mental health challenges. LLMs can assist therapists by offering insights or by acting as supplementary tools between sessions, providing continuous patient engagement. In motivational interviewing, LLMs can help patients reflect on their thoughts and behaviors, encouraging them to make positive changes in their lives. By offering accessible, round-the-clock support, LLMs help enhance patient engagement in mental health treatment, making therapy more accessible and personalized. A study [76] states that automatically coding patient behaviors is essential for supporting psychotherapists' decision-making during Motivational Interviewing (MI), an interactive communication approach used to address psychiatric issues such as alcohol and drug addiction. While in the past, the task of coding behavior has used machine learning to predict patients' status during MI sessions, the lack of specific domain knowledge and the disregard of patient-therapist interactions are the main challenges in the development and use of these models in practice and the real world. The authors introduce the Chain-of-Interaction (CoI) method to address these challenges, aiming to contextualize large language models to support psychiatric decision-making through dual interactions. The CoI approach systematically divides the coding task into four key stages: reasoning, extracting patient interaction, learning therapist question strategies, and integrating dual interactions between patients and therapists. This method allows large language models to use the coding scheme, patient status, and domain knowledge to code patient behavior. Experiments on real datasets demonstrated the effective-ness and flexibility of the authors' proposed method with several advanced LLM models compared to existing baselines in the field of stimulation. Additionally, the authors conducted extensive analysis and demonstrated the critical role of dual interactions in applying LLMs to understand psychotherapy behavior. Experiments were also conducted on four LLMs, namely Llama2-13B-Chat [64], Falcon-7B-Instruct [77], Mistral-7B-Instruct [78] and Chat-GPT, which are available through the OpenAI API2[2] or Hugging Face3.[3] The reason for choosing these LLMs over their untuned base versions (e.g., Llama2-13B-Base, Falcon-7B-Base) is their superior ability to follow conversational-style instructions. Finally, using a real dataset of motivational interviews, the proposed Chain-of-Interaction invocation method was compared with four advanced large language models. The results show that this method achieved superior performance. The authors conducted an ablation analysis, which showed that removing any stage from the Chain-of-Interaction leads to a significant reduction in performance. As a result, this experiment demonstrated the effectiveness of each stage.

2.2.3 LLMs for Medical Text Summarization

LLMs have the capability to summarize complex medical texts, making it easier for patients and healthcare professionals to understand vast amounts of clinical data. By converting lengthy medical reports, research papers, or patient records into digestible summaries, LLMs support patients in better understanding their health conditions, treatment options, and prognosis. For healthcare providers, this enhances communication, enabling more informed decision-making and improving the overall patient experience. LLM-powered summarization tools ensure that patients remain engaged in their healthcare journey by simplifying medical information, which is often a barrier to patient understanding and participation. The study [79] focuses on evaluating the performance of two open-source large language models, Llama2-70B and Mistral-7B, in summarizing three types of medical conversations, assessing them on relevant datasets: MEDIQA-QS [80], MeQSum [81], MEDIQA-ANS [82], MEDIQA-MAS [80] and iCliniq [83]. The goal of this study is to explore the capability and quality of using open-source large language models for extractive and abstractive summarization of medical conversations, which is useful for supporting clinical decision-making, patient education, and summarizing medical records. It is important to note that this area remains a new and active field of research, with many aspects related to validity and reliability still unclear. The unique innovation and contribution of this approach lies in the use of a target model as a comparative reference, aiming to reduce the total number of pairwise comparisons and minimize associated time and costs. For each test sample, summaries

[2] https://platform.openai.com/docs/guides/gpt/chat-completions-api

[3] https://huggingface.co

generated by the two open-source large language models are presented to GPT-4, which is asked to compare them against a summary generated by GPT-3.5 across four key dimensions: relevance (selection of key information), coherence (logical flow and transitions), fluency (grammatical correctness and readability), and factuality (accurate alignment with the input). GPT-4 selects the best summary for each pair and briefly explains its reasons for the selection. This pairwise comparison is repeated with the order of summaries swapped to avoid positional bias Initial results on a subset of test data indicate that Llama2 outperforms Mistral in most evaluation dimensions across the three datasets. Overall, this study provides a solution to the critical need for systematic evaluation and comparison of large language models in the context of medical text summarization tasks. The authors' proposed evaluation approach, using GPT-4 as the evaluator, can enable quality control, support the selection of effective large language models for specific tasks, and advance knowledge discovery in digital health. As open-source large language models continue to evolve, their potential for medical text summarization increases. However, rigorous evaluation, domain alignment, and integration with human expertise will be crucial to ensure the reliability, safety, and utility of medical summaries generated by large language models in real-world clinical applications [71].

2.2.4 Sentiment Analysis of Patient Reviews Using Hybrid Models

Sentiment analysis, powered by LLMs, is an invaluable tool for assessing patient feedback and reviews. LLMs can efficiently analyze patient reviews, extracting insights regarding patient satisfaction, concerns, and areas needing improvement. This type of analysis enables healthcare providers to better understand the emotional tone behind patient experiences, providing actionable data to enhance service quality and engagement strategies. By identifying patterns in patient sentiment, healthcare organizations can proactively address patient needs, tailoring their services to improve patient trust, satisfaction, and engagement. This promotes a more patient-centered approach to healthcare and helps organizations make data-driven decisions to improve the patient experience. The study [84] states that with the advancement of internet technology and its increasing penetration in various parts of the world, the number of internet users and e-commerce platforms has grown significantly. To help doctors understand patients' mental states and provide better diagnoses and treatments, all major hospitals and online medical platforms offer review sections to display patient opinions based on their previous medical experiences. By collecting and interpreting the text of published reviews for sentiment analysis, users can view the real opinions of other users about doctors and hospitals, and doctors and hospitals can receive direct feedback from patients. However, as the volume of textual review data accumulates, it becomes difficult to extract effective information due to the sheer amount of data, and the sentiment trends derived from traditional analysis algorithms are relatively vague. Therefore, quickly identifying the overall sentiment of review texts and accurately analyzing sentiment trends across all aspects of the reviews is crucial. This study proposes a hybrid model of

BERT and TextCNN to extract emotional features and analyze sentiment information in the reviews. Experimental results on a dataset of medical reviews show that this method performs well. This study helps improve the understanding of patients' true emotions and can positively impact patient engagement and the quality of medical services.

In a similar study [85], the critical role of emotional context in patient-doctor conversations is examined. Comprehensive sentiment analysis was conducted using advanced deep learning models, including BERT, RoBERTa, GPT-2, and XLNet. The dataset used comprised 185 hours of Greek conversations related to hematologic malignancies. The study's methodology included data collection, data labeling, model training, and performance evaluation using metrics such as accuracy, precision, recall, F1 score, and specificity. The results showed that BERT outperformed other methods in all emotional categories, demonstrating high effectiveness in understanding emotional context in clinical interactions. RoBERTa showed strong performance in identifying neutral emotions. GPT-2 produced promising results for neutral emotions but had lower precision and recall for negative emotions. XLNet had moderate performance with variability across different categories. The authors' findings highlight the complexities of sentiment analysis in clinical settings, especially in less commonly used languages like Greek. These results emphasize the potential of advanced deep learning models to improve communication and patient care in healthcare environments. Integrating sentiment analysis into healthcare can provide valuable insights into patients' emotional states, leading to more effective and empathetic support for patients.

2.2.5 Analyzing Patient Experience Data

LLMs offer advanced capabilities for analyzing patient experience data, such as feedback from surveys, reviews, or social media interactions. These models can identify trends, pinpoint concerns, and help healthcare providers understand how patients perceive various aspects of care. By using LLMs to analyze large-scale data, healthcare organizations can better respond to patient preferences and concerns, ultimately improving the overall care experience. This form of analysis contributes directly to patient engagement by enabling more personalized and responsive healthcare strategies, ensuring that patients feel heard and that their feedback is valued in shaping their healthcare experience. The study [86], the authors state that with the increasing focus of healthcare systems on care quality and patient-centered care, patient perspectives on the services provided have become an essential part of healthcare service evaluations. Patient experiences can be used to improve care quality, as they offer valuable insights into interactions with healthcare services. An increasing number of organizations systematically collect and analyze patient experience data. The aim of this study was to identify key themes in patient experiences related to healthcare and analyze readers' reactions to these experiences. In this study, 1663 blogs and 298,806 textual comments about adverse patient experiences were extracted from a Hungarian online forum over a 10-year period. Topic modeling was used with advanced BERT tokens to analyze the data and extract meaningful patterns and concepts. Sentiment analysis was used to categorize the emotional intensity of the narrative writings. The huBERT and HIL-SBERT models identified 326 and 200 topics related to patient experiences and 508 and 728 topics related to reactions to these experiences, respectively, without human supervision. Concep-tually similar topics were manually merged into main categories. 94.4% of the experiences and 77.5% of the comments were classified as negative, showing the same annual trend over a decade. This study uses a data-driven approach to extract patterns from patient comments in the context of healthcare in Hungary. Topic modeling based on BERT tokens can provide valuable insights into patient perceptions and views, which can help improve the quality and safety of healthcare.

In another study [87], the focus is on the limitations of traditional prescribed dietary programs, which are often lacking in personalization and difficult to follow. The authors propose an innovative approach that utilizes generative AI within a learning health system framework, with a focus on clinical nutrition for hospitalized patients. This system includes two key models: the Meal Image Generation Model (MealIGM), and the Meal Plan Generation Model (MealImageGM), which leverage advanced large language models. The MealIGM model gradually improves by using patient information from electronic health records and clinical nutrition guidelines, with feedback from dietitians and users. On the other hand, the MealImageGM model generates images of meal plans to increase patient engagement and help optimize image generation requests based on collected feedback. The overall process of the system involves extracting data from electronic health records, designing pre-set meal requests for users, and generating personalized meal plans and images. Dietitians play a crucial role in monitoring patient adherence and preferences, contributing to the system's continuous learning cycle. The proposed framework ensures that meal plans are clinically appropriate, perso-nalized, and aligned with dynamic dietary recommendations. This study emphasizes the importance of patient and physician collaboration for ongoing optimization and highlights the potential positive impact on health outcomes.

2.2.6 ChatGPT's Role in Enhancing Diabetes Care and Patient Engagement

ChatGPT, as an example of an LLM, can play a significant role in enhancing diabetes care and patient engagement. By offering personalized health advice, reminders for medication adherence, and interactive support, ChatGPT can keep patients actively involved in managing their diabetes. The model can educate patients on lifestyle changes, provide tips on diet and exercise, and answer common queries related to diabetes management. ChatGPT can also be integrated into diabetes monitoring apps, offering real-time support and feedback based on patient data. Its ability to deliver tailored, empathetic interactions helps build patient trust, making them more engaged and proactive in their care. In another study [88], the authors focus on adding sentiment labels to free-text comments in patient surveys collected by the

Norwegian Institute of Public Health (NIPH). Labeling these comments can be time-consuming and resource-intensive, especially when domain expertise is required. In this study, in addition to manual labeling, a potential alternative to human labeling is explored by using large language models as labelers. Two pre-trained large language models for the Norwegian language were evaluated, and various settings of prompts and in-context learning were tested. The results show that even in zero-shot scenarios, these models significantly outperformed the baseline in binary sentiment analysis. However, these models still cannot compete with human labelers when analyzing complete datasets. This research emphasizes the importance of using large language models in sentiment analysis and suggests that these techniques can serve as helpful tools to enhance the process of analyzing patient comments, although they do not yet match the accuracy and quality of human analyses.

In another study [89], the authors aim to shed light on the transformative potential of large language models like ChatGPT in enhancing diabetes care by presenting a new approach. The main focus of the authors' discussion is ChatGPT's ability to enhance patient engagement, provide personalized medical guidance, and improve workflows in healthcare. They suggest that ChatGPT could be a pivotal technology capable of transforming traditional patterns in diabetes management and patient care. Personalization is at the forefront of modern healthcare innovations. ChatGPT's adaptive learning capabilities allow it to offer personalized recommendations and information to individuals with diabetes. This means that patients can receive customized educational content aligned with their unique health status and learning preferences, thereby boosting their ability to manage and navigate their condition with confidence and informed independence. Moreover, ChatGPT can analyze patient preferences, blood glucose control data, and current dietary guidelines, as well as dietitian recommend-ations, to create personalized meal plans and provide real-time feedback for optimizing blood sugar control. Additionally, the integration of ChatGPT with Continuous Glucose Monitoring (CGM) systems can enhance its ability to offer timely and tailored dietary recommendations, potentially improving diabetes self-management. The study also highlights ChatGPT's application in mental health care, pointing to its broader potential to provide emotional support across various healthcare domains, including diabetes care. ChatGPT facilitates a more personalized interaction, which can be beneficial in offering emotional support to those struggling with diabetes. Furthermore, ChatGPT can be used to generate appropriate medication reminders, explain medication instructions, and provide real-time feedback on adherence. Its conversational interface can create a user-friendly environment for individuals to discuss their medication regimen, seek clarification, and be encouraged to adhere to their treatment plans. The integration of ChatGPT with existing digital health platforms could potentially enhance the effectiveness of medication reminders and adherence strategies, particularly in the self-management of diabetes. However, the authors emphasize that further research is necessary to evaluate the effectiveness, user acceptance, and ethical considerations of using ChatGPT in this critical aspect of diabetes care. Ultimately, ChatGPT is poised to emerge as a powerful ally in diabetes care, offering immediate support by providing instant responses to diabetes-related queries, thereby enhancing the accessibility and responsiveness of patient support mechanisms.

2.2.7 Advancements in AI-Driven Medical Diagnostics and Patient Support

The advancements in AI-driven diagnostics, powered by LLMs, are revolutionizing how patients engage with their healthcare. LLMs can assist in early diagnosis by interpreting medical records, lab results, and imaging data, helping clinicians identify potential health issues with greater accuracy and speed. These models also provide patients with more immediate, understandable feedback about their health, allowing them to be more informed and involved in their care decisions. Additionally, AI-powered support tools can assist patients in managing chronic diseases, scheduling appointments, and providing follow-up care instructions. This fosters a more engaged and empowered patient, who feels actively involved in their healthcare journey. In study [90], the integration of disease knowledge with BERT models to improve key health-related tasks has been proposed. Specifically, a novel method for training disease knowledge integration has been introduced and evaluated on a range of BERT models, including BERT, BioBERT, SciBERT, ClinicalBERT, BlueBERT, and ALBERT. Experiments on three different tasks show that these models can improve in most cases, indicating the feasibility of integrating disease knowledge. For example, the accuracy of the BioBERT model in answering consumer health questions increased from 68.29% to 72.09%, and new results were observed in two datasets. This research suggests that integrating disease knowledge with advanced language models can significantly enhance their performance in answering health-related questions and other related tasks. In another study [91], the authors state that medical images play a crucial role in the medical field, and an advanced system for answering visual medical questions could assist in disease diagnosis. However, no entirely satisfactory method has been proposed to comprehensively solve this problem so far. In this study, a model called CGMVQA is proposed, which aims to convert this complex problem into several simpler tasks, incorporating classification and answer generation capabilities. Various techniques have been used to optimize this model. For instance, data augmentation has been applied to images to increase data diversity, and text tokenization has been performed for optimal processing of textual information. Visual features were extracted using the pre-trained ResNet152 model, and three different types of embeddings were used for text processing. Additionally, reducing the parameters of the multihead self-attention transformer to lower computational costs and tuning the masking and output layers for model performance optimization were carried out. The CGMVQA model achieved new results on the ImageCLEF 2019 VQA-Med datasets, with a classification accuracy of 0.640, word match score of 0.659, and semantic similarity score of 0.678. These results demonstrate the capability of the CGMVQA model in answering visual medical questions, indicating that this model could effectively assist physicians in clinical analyses and disease diagnosis.

Additionally, in study [50], the authors explore how generative visual question-answering systems can responsibly support patients' informational needs in the context of radiology imaging data. In this research, a preliminary study was conducted in which participants reviewed chest computed tomography (CT) scans and the associated radiology reports of a hypothetical relative and engaged in a discussion with a cardiothoracic radiologist. Through thematic analysis of the conversations between the participants and medical professionals, common themes were identified, including the explanation of medical terms, identification of issues mentioned in the report within the scanned image, understanding the disease prognosis, discussing subsequent diagnostic steps, and comparing treatment options. Based on these themes, two advanced generative visual language models were compared with the radiologists' responses. The results indicated variability in the quality of the answers generated by the models across different topics. This study highlights the importance of patient-centered generative AI systems that can cover a wide range of conversational topics and meet the real informational needs of patients.

Lastly, it should be noted that the lack of transparency and interpretability of large language models, especially for critical and irreversible medical decision-making, poses a significant challenge. The study [92] suggests that to better utilize these models, there is a need to enhance their "explainability." This refers to the need to understand the internal workings of these models to comprehend how they arrived at a specific output. This need for "explainability" in machine learning models has led to the emergence of a branch of interpretable artificial intelligence, recently known as "eXplainable Artificial Intelligence" or XAI.

2.3 *Innovative Approaches to Enhancing Patient Interaction and Engagement with AI*

In the previous sections of the chapter, various aspects of generative AI were discussed, including GANs and LLMs. This section explores other innovative approaches in patient interaction. These approaches include new methods and complementary technologies that help improve patient-doctor communications and create new potentials for enhancing patient experiences. By analyzing these methods, this section examines how different technologies can be combined to increase patient engagement and interaction in treatment processes.

2.3.1 Mobile Applications and Virtual Assistants

The study [93], states that generative AI can facilitate seamless communication between patients and providers, enhancing both patient engagement and understanding. Through natural language processing and conversational AI, patients can access personalized health information, receive appropriate education, and participate in virtual consultations, reinforcing a patient-centered approach to healthcare. This study introduces two patient engagement tools as follows:

- Mobile Applications: Designing mobile apps with personalized health insights, appointment reminders, medication tracking, and telehealth features to engage patients in self-care and treatment adherence.
- Chatbots and Virtual Assistants: Introducing AI-powered chatbots and virtual assistants for real-time communication, answering patient questions, providing education, and guiding patients through treatment plans.

The study also mentions that generative AI has significantly improved patient communication and interaction. By using natural language processing, AI systems provide clear and understandable explanations of medical conditions and treatment plans, leading to better patient comprehension of their health scenarios. Approximately 78% of patients reported a better understanding of their conditions and treatment options. Moreover, AI-facilitated virtual mental health services, combining cognitive-behavioral therapy techniques and mindfulness practices, have shown significant improvements in users' mental well-being. As a result, integrating generative AI into healthcare and patient services represents a transformative step forward in the medical field, bringing unprecedented levels of personalization, efficiency, and patient engagement. This technology has demonstrated that by using AI to develop appropriate treatment plans and lifestyle recommendations, healthcare providers can significantly improve patient adherence to treatments and overall health outcomes. The ability to customize care to fit patient profiles marks a paradigm shift toward more preventive and patient-centered care.

2.3.2 Wearable Technologies and Patient-Computer Interfaces

In another study [94], the authors state that since patients' bodies and dialysis machines work together, there is an inevitable connection between them. Additionally, data from wearable technologies (including variables such as heart rate, sleep, physical activity, electro-cardiography, oxygen saturation, and glucose monitoring) and self-reported questionnaires via smartphones provide insights into the application, usability, and relevance of technology in daily human life, especially in designing user-centered technology and developing the Internet of Things. These can play an important role in personalized medicine. Therefore, the development of a Patient-Computer Interface (PPCI) in dialysis, aiming to integrate computer technology and patient-specific data into the management of dialysis treatment, enhances the patient experience by providing a personalized and interactive interface. This interface allows patients to take a more active role in their dialysis treatment, as updated information about their health status, symptoms, and preferences can be used to tailor dialysis treatment according to their specific needs. A personalized approach can help optimize treatment outcomes and improve patient satisfaction. Moreover, PPCI can offer educational materials and interactive tools to monitor treatment progress and provide real-time feedback on health status, thereby improving patient engagement and self-care. The most common human-computer interaction technologies currently in use fall under the concept of mHealth.[4] The potential of wearable sensor data for predicting laboratory results and remote patient monitoring has been highlighted. For instance, combining environmental sensors (such as depth cameras and microphones) with wearable data can improve the reliability of fall detection systems while keeping the false alarm rate low. Consequently, the number of studies using digital products is rapidly increasing. In this context, integrating a conversational LLM AI like ChatGPT with PPCI should further enhance the patient experience by offering natural language interaction, enabling patients to ask questions about dialysis, receive personalized recommendations, and get support for any concerns about their treatments [94].

2.3.3 Generative Co-design Frameworks and Cost Savings

Finally, the study [95] provides a generative co-design framework for healthcare innovators seeking to expand their innovations beyond the pilot stage, offering guidance on incorporating the end user's voice in the design of healthcare innovations. This framework contributes to the literature on patient engagement by presenting a new category of patient engagement framework that focuses on involving end-users in the creative process of healthcare innovation. Healthcare innovators, applied health sciences researchers, clinicians, and quality improvement professionals may refer to the framework and case study presented here to extract practical considerations for healthcare innovation and design. Additionally, in the study [96], the authors state that from the provider's perspective, Generative AI can save costs by simplifying administrative tasks, improving efficiency, early disease detection, and preventive care. Similarly, understanding the initial evidence of using Generative AI across healthcare services is crucial for making informed decisions, ensuring regulatory compliance, building trust, guiding research initiatives, and addressing ethical considerations. This lays the foundation for the responsible and effective integration of Generative AI into the healthcare landscape.

3 Applications of Generative AI in Patient Engagement

Generative AI in patient engagement has widespread applications. This approach leverages the power of generative AI to significantly enhance patient interactions, leading to improved health outcomes and more personalized care. The following are the applications and practical uses in this area:

[4] Mobile Health (mHealth) delivers healthcare services through smartphones, allowing users to manage their wellbeing, access medical information, and receive tailored health advice.

3.1 Appointment Management with Consultants and Physicians

In today's world, people are often unwilling to go to hospitals and wait in line for consultations with doctors [97]. Patients do not want to waste time, effort, and money waiting at the hospital reception [97]. A study [98] states that AI chatbots have revolutionized the way appointments are scheduled and managed. A patient can interact with a chatbot through a clinic's website or a mobile app to schedule their appointment. Using natural language processing, the chatbot understands the patient's request and suggests available times by accessing the clinic's scheduling system. This system not only saves time for both the patient and administrative staff but also reduces the likelihood of common errors associated with manual scheduling.

3.2 Predictive Modeling for Personalized Treatment

Integrating AI into the healthcare sector has the potential to transform human suffering and enhance performance and outcomes from disease diagnosis to specific treatment plans [99]. Generative AI can analyze patients' health records and lifestyle information to provide personalized health tips [98]. Predictive models based on generative AI can anticipate patients' reactions to various treatment options. By simulating different scenarios, these models help health professionals select the most effective and safest treatment methods for each patient, resulting in improved treatment outcomes and increased patient satisfaction. This approach enables doctors to make more precise decisions and choose treatments with the highest chances of success, tailored to each patient's specific needs. This approach is an effective step towards personalizing treatments and overall improvement in healthcare delivery. For example, a diabetic patient may receive appropriate dietary recommendations and exercise tips based on their latest glucose levels and physical activity data [98].

3.3 Integration of Diverse Data Sources

Modern healthcare systems need to monitor temporal changes, manage key features, and provide robust search capabilities that go beyond electronic health records [100]. Generative AI possesses the unique ability to integrate and analyze diverse data sources, including test results, medical histories, imaging data, and patient statements. This comprehensive analysis provides a complete view of the patient's health status and allows for the development of personalized treatment plans that consider all aspects of the patient's condition. As a result, the treatments provided are not only more effective but also more aligned with the specific conditions and needs of each patient. This advanced approach can make significant changes, especially in complex treatments and patients with multiple chronic diseases.

3.4 Increased Access and Ease

A study [98] states that generative AI significantly improves access to communications in healthcare. AI-based systems such as chatbots and virtual assistants are not limited to office hours and provide 24-hour support to patients. This continuous access is especially beneficial for patients who may need help outside regular working hours. For example, a patient experiencing medication side effects in the middle of the night can receive immediate guidance from an AI assistant, which can reduce the patient's anxiety and prevent unnecessary emergency room visits [98]. Furthermore, it is important to note that patients' interest in and ability to use patient portals are heavily influenced by personal factors such as age, ethnicity, education level, health literacy, health status, and caregiver role [101].

3.5 Virtual Health Assistants

Inadequate patient care in healthcare systems is a key issue that leads to lower patient satisfaction and increased medical errors [102]. Virtual healthcare assistants, such as ChatGPT, have emerged as a promising solution to mitigate these challenges [102]. Figure 5 illustrates how a generative AI-based digital assistant can provide patients with the necessary information and guidance. A study [103]. indicates that virtual health assistants powered by generative AI play a significant role in improving patient interaction with healthcare systems. These assistants not only answer patient questions but also provide regular medication reminders, helping patients stay on track with their treatment. This feature is particularly important for patients with chronic conditions who require ongoing and precise management of their treatment. By using these virtual assistants, patients can easily access medical information and advice, and quickly receive guidance if any concerns arise or immediate consultation is needed.

Additionally, virtual health assistants can offer valuable assistance in emergency situations [103]. These assistants can analyze patients' symptoms and provide immediate and appropriate advice for the patient's condition. This capability allows patients to benefit from healthcare services promptly without needing to visit healthcare facilities in person. As a result, virtual health assistants can help reduce the burden on healthcare facilities, increase patient satisfaction, and improve treatment outcomes. This technology not only facilitates access to healthcare but also significantly enhances the quality and efficiency of these services [103]. Furthermore, these assistants can send personalized reminders to patients to take their medications according to their specific schedules. These reminders can include educational

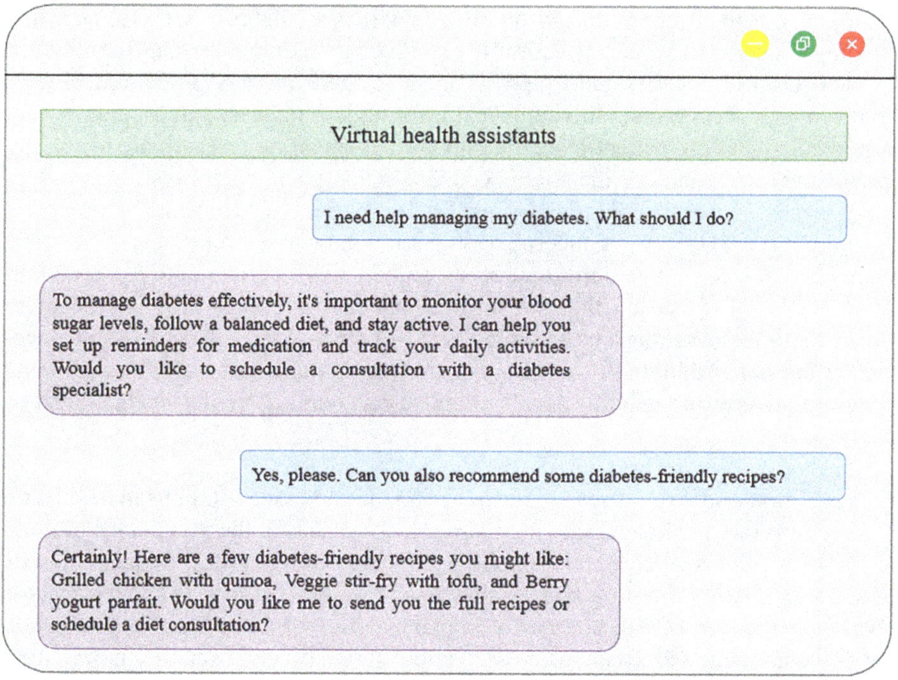

Fig. 5 A generative AI-based digital assistant providing patients with the information and guidance they need

content about the importance of adherence and the effectiveness of the medication, thus promoting better understanding and compliance [98].

4 Challenges and Limitations

In the healthcare sector, the integration of generative AI presents numerous challenges and future directions that shape its potential impact on patient care and clinical performance. Addressing these challenges and outlining future paths to maximize the benefits of generative AI while minimizing potential risks and ensuring responsible use is essential. These challenges include the need for high-quality, large-volume data, model complexity, and heavy computational requirements. Additionally, issues related to inaccurate or incomplete data, ethical concerns, data privacy, and the lack of trust and acceptance by patients toward these models are other barriers facing this field.

Data Privacy and Security: Ensuring patient privacy and adhering to regulatory standards while developing personalized treatments add layers of complexity. Ensuring compliance with data protection laws, maintaining patient privacy, obtaining informed consent, and addressing issues of liability are complex and ongoing concerns that must be carefully examined to maintain trust and confidence in AI-based healthcare systems [104]. The use of generative AI in patient interactions requires access to sensitive medical information. Increased transparency and, in particular, sharing patient-level data for further scientific research are becoming increasingly important for the pharmaceutical industry and other organizations that support and conduct clinical trials, as well as for the benefit of patients participating in studies [105]. However, concerns remain about how to appropriately collect and share clinical trial data with third-party researchers while maintaining patient confidentiality [105]. Ensuring that patient data are properly encrypted and securely stored requires investment in advanced security technologies and robust management processes. Additionally, gaining patient trust in the use of their data within AI systems and ensuring that this data is not misused are other challenges that must be addressed.

Patient Trust and Acceptance: The adoption of innovative solutions in healthcare continues to face challenges, adding to broader obstacles in the acceptance of these technologies in both private and public healthcare settings [106]. Patients may be hesitant to trust AI due to a lack of understanding of how it works and concerns about potential errors. The successful implementation of AI in healthcare relies on the understanding and acceptance of its applications by end-users, including both medical professionals and patients. This understanding fosters trust in AI systems, enabling effective use and gradually addressing ethical and regulatory challenges [107]. Building trust among patients and ensuring that the results and recommendations provided by AI are reliable are other significant challenges.

Interpretation and Explainability of Results: One of the challenges of generative AI is the explainability of its results. The lack of interpretability and explainability in generative AI models creates difficulties in understanding how AI-driven decisions are made [105]. In clinical environments where transparency and accountability are priorities, the opaque nature of AI models can hinder trust and acceptance among healthcare providers and patients [105]. A study [108] highlights a major risk of AI: it can be perceived as a "black box," limiting trust in its reliability, which is a critical issue in a field where decisions can mean the difference between life and death. As a result, the concept of Explainable AI (XAI) is gaining traction. XAI aims to ensure that AI algorithms (and the decisions they produce) are understandable to humans. Consequently, transparency and explainability in this space must be carefully considered to prevent unforeseen consequences.

Data Quality: Access to high-quality and diverse data is essential for training accurate and efficient AI models. In the healthcare sector, data is often fragmented and stored across various systems, making comprehensive and complete data difficult to access for AI model development [108]. Collecting and integrating this data poses significant challenges, especially considering privacy concerns, the need for data security, and compliance with legal regulations. Additionally, data quality is a major concern, as incorrect or insufficient data can lead to the development of inaccurate and ineffective models. The more data that is publicly accessible, the greater the transparency of the results.

Model Bias: Bias refers to systematic errors in decision-making processes that result in unfair outcomes [109]. Identifying and addressing bias in AI is crucial to ensuring that these systems are fair and equitable for all users [109]. Generative AI models produce outputs based on training data derived from medical records and scientific literature. If this data contains biases, the generated results will also be flawed [110]. Models trained on large, unfiltered internet data, such as ChatGPT or Steady Diffusion, are at risk of repeating, amplifying, and spreading negative and inaccurate content due to the mix of correct and incorrect information, biases, and both harmful and harmless content they absorb [110]. To mitigate the effects of bias, training data should be carefully selected, AI models must be fine-tuned with precision, and continuous evaluation and review processes should be implemented. Establishing strong ethical and legal frameworks for AI and machine learning systems is essential to ensure that privacy, transparency, and accountability are not just peripheral issues, but fundamental elements throughout the AI development cycle [109].

5 Conclusion

In this chapter, the role of generative artificial intelligence in enhancing patient engagement was examined. Patient engagement is recognized as a critical element in improving the quality of healthcare. With its advanced and innovative capabilities, generative AI can elevate this engagement to a new level, leading to increased patient satisfaction. By reviewing various patient engagement models based on generative AI, it was demonstrated that this technology can strengthen interactions between patients and healthcare systems, creating new opportunities for enhancing healthcare services. These innovations not only empower patients with greater control over their health but also simplify workflows for healthcare professionals. However, challenges such as data quality, algorithmic biases, and ethical and legal issues, which could negatively impact the implementation of these technologies, were also discussed. Therefore, while the applications of generative AI in the healthcare sector are vast and can bring significant improvements in quality and efficiency, existing challenges must be addressed, and strong ethical and legal frameworks must be established to fully harness this technology. Ultimately, generative AI has the potential to overcome current challenges and serve as a powerful tool for increasing patient engagement and improving the quality of healthcare. It is anticipated that in the future, researchers and scientists will be able to create models in which healthcare is not just about treating and caring for patients, but about empowering and engaging individuals to lead healthier and more fulfilling lives. By embracing the potential of generative AI in the medical field, we can broaden our perspectives and understanding, ultimately increasing patient satisfaction.

References

1. Bachina L, Kanagala A. Health revolution: AI-powered patient engagement. J Chem Biochem Sci. 2023;24(5)
2. Moglia A, Georgiou K, Georgiou E, Satava RM, Cuschieri A. A systematic review on artificial intelligence in robot-assisted surgery. Int J Surg. 2021;95:106151.
3. Payrovnaziri SN, et al. Explainable artificial intelligence models using real-world electronic health record data: a systematic scoping review. J Am Med Inform Assoc. 2020;27(7):1173–85.
4. Shaik T, et al. Remote patient monitoring using artificial intelligence: current state, applications, and challenges. Wiley Interdiscip Rev Data Min Knowl Discov. 2023;13(2):e1485.
5. Khan ZF, Alotaibi SR. Applications of artificial intelligence and big data analytics in m-health: a healthcare system perspective. J Healthc Eng. 2020;2020(1):8894694.
6. Yu H, Zhou Z. Optimization of IoT-based artificial intelligence assisted telemedicine health analysis system. IEEE Access. 2021;9:85034–48.
7. Alowais SA, et al. Revolutionizing healthcare: the role of artificial intelligence in clinical practice. BMC Med Educ. 2023;23(1):689.
8. Marzban S, Najafi M, Agolli A, Ashrafi E. Impact of patient engagement on healthcare quality: a scoping review. J Patient Exp. 2022;9:23743735221125440.
9. Graffigna G, Barello S, Wiederhold BK, Bosio AC, Riva G. Positive technology as a driver for health engagement. Annu Rev Cyberther Telemed. 2013;2013:9–17.
10. Stewart R, Liabo K. Involvement in research without compromising research quality. J Health Serv Res Policy. 2012;17(4):248–51.
11. Habicht J, Dina LM, Stylianou M, Harper R, Hauser TU, Rollwage M. Generative AI-enabled therapy support tool improves clinical outcomes and patient engagement in NHS talking therapies; 2024.
12. Davis K, Schoenbaum SC, Audet A-M. A 2020 vision of patient-centered primary care. J Gen Intern Med. 2005;20:953–7.
13. Barello S, et al. eHealth for patient engagement: a systematic review. Front Psychol. 2016;6:2013.
14. Schwappach DLB, Wernli M. Am I (un) safe here? Chemotherapy patients' perspectives towards engaging in their safety. Qual Saf Health Care. 2010;19(5):e9.
15. Gallivan J, Kovacs Burns K, Bellows M, Eigenseher C. The many faces of patient engagement. J Particip Med. 2012;4(23):e32.
16. Haywood K, Lyddiatt A, Brace-McDonnell SJ, Staniszewska S, Salek S. Establishing the values for patient engagement (PE) in health-related quality of life (HRQoL) research: an international, multiple-stakeholder perspective. Qual Life Res. 2017;26:1393–404.
17. Chafe R, Levinson W, Hébert PC. The need for public engagement in choosing health priorities. Can Med Assoc. 2011;183:165.
18. Barello S, Graffigna G, Vegni E, Bosio AC. The challenges of conceptualizing patient engagement in health care: a lexicographic literature review. J Particip Med. 2014;6(11):259–67.
19. Manafo E, Petermann L, Mason-Lai P, Vandall-Walker V. Patient engagement in Canada: a scoping review of the 'how'and 'what'of patient engagement in health research. Health Res Policy Syst. 2018;16:1–11.
20. Street RL Jr, Millay B. Analyzing patient participation in medical encounters. Health Commun. 2001;13(1):61–73.
21. Carman KL, et al. Patient and family engagement: a framework for understanding the elements and developing interventions and policies. Health Aff. 2013;32(2):223–31.
22. Graffigna G, Barello S, Bonanomi A, Lozza E. Measuring patient engagement: development and psychometric properties of the Patient Health Engagement (PHE) Scale. Front Psychol. 2015;6:274.
23. Domecq JP, et al. Patient engagement in research: a systematic review. BMC Health Serv Res. 2014;14:1–9.

24. Abma TA, Broerse JEW. Patient participation as dialogue: setting research agendas. Health Expect. 2010;13(2):160–73.
25. Frank L, et al. Conceptual and practical foundations of patient engagement in research at the patient-centered outcomes research institute. Qual Life Res. 2015;24:1033–41.
26. Menichetti J, Libreri C, Lozza E, Graffigna G. Giving patients a starring role in their own care: a bibliometric analysis of the on-going literature debate. Health Expect. 2016;19(3):516–26.
27. Gandhi P. Transformation in healthcare industry to boost patient engagement using AI. J Informatics Educ Res. 2024;4(2)
28. Lysen F, Wyatt S. Refusing participation: hesitations about designing responsible patient engagement with artificial intelligence in healthcare. J Responsib Innov. 2024;11(1):2300161.
29. Bareis J, Katzenbach C. Talking AI into being: the narratives and imaginaries of national AI strategies and their performative politics. Sci Technol Hum Values. 2022;47(5):855–81.
30. Maslej N, et al. Artificial intelligence index report 2023. arXiv preprint arXiv. 2023:2310.03715.
31. Seyyed-Kalantari L, Zhang H, McDermott MBA, Chen IY, Ghassemi M. Underdiagnosis bias of artificial intelligence algorithms applied to chest radiographs in under-served patient populations. Nat Med. 2021;27(12):2176–82.
32. Ackermans L, Hageman MG, Bos AH, Haverkamp D, Scholtes VAB, Poolman RW. Feedback to patients about patient-reported outcomes does not improve empowerment or satisfaction. Clin Orthop Relat Res. 2018;476(4):716–22.
33. Aradau C, Bunz M. Dismantling the apparatus of domination?: left critiques of AI. Radic Philos. 2022;212:10–8.
34. Shaw J, Sekalala S. Health data justice: building new norms for health data governance. NPJ Digit Med. 2023;6(1):30.
35. Powles J, Hodson H. Google DeepMind and healthcare in an age of algorithms. Health Technol (Berl). 2017;7(4):351–67.
36. Wilson C. Public engagement and AI: a values analysis of national strategies. Gov Inf Q. 2022;39(1):101652.
37. WHO. Patient engagement: elevating the voices of patients and families for safer care. Accessed 24 Aug 2024. [Online]. Available: https://www.who.int/westernpacific/news-room/feature-stories/item/patient-engagement%2D%2Delevating-the-voices-of-patients-and-families-for-safer-care
38. Del Savio L, Prainsack B, Buyx A. Motivations of participants in the citizen science of microbiomics: data from the British Gut Project. Genet Med. 2017;19(8):959–61.
39. Clavel N, Badr J, Gautier L, Lavoie-Tremblay M, Paquette J. Risk perceptions, knowledge and behaviors of general and high-risk adult populations towards COVID-19: a systematic scoping review. Public Health Rev. 2021;42:1603979.
40. Feuerriegel S, Hartmann J, Janiesch C, Zschech P. Generative ai. Bus Inf Syst Eng. 2024;66(1):111–26.
41. Bandi A, Adapa PVSR, Kuchi YEVPK. The power of generative ai: a review of requirements, models, input–output formats, evaluation metrics, and challenges. Fut Internet. 2023;15(8):260.
42. Sehrawat SK. Empowering the patient journey: the role of generative AI in healthcare. Int J Sustain Dev Through AI ML IoT. 2023;2(2):1–18.
43. Fui-Hoon Nah F, Zheng R, Cai J, Siau K, Chen L. Generative AI and ChatGPT: applications, challenges, and AI-human collaboration, vol. 25. Taylor & Francis; 2023. p. 277–304.
44. Saxena D, Cao J. Generative adversarial networks (GANs) challenges, solutions, and future directions. ACM Comput Surv (CSUR). 2021;54(3):1–42.
45. Alqahtani H, Kavakli-Thorne M, Kumar G. Applications of generative adversarial networks (gans): an updated review. Arch Comput Methods Eng. 2021;28:525–52.
46. Saaran V, Kushwaha V, Gupta S, Agarwal G. A literature review on generative adversarial networks with its applications in healthcare. In: Congress on intelligent systems. Springer; 2020. p. 215–25.

47. Bhatt C, Bhatia A. Generative adversarial networks applications. RES MILITARIS. 2020;10(1):105–11.
48. Wang L, Chen W, Yang W, Bi F, Yu FR. A state-of-the-art review on image synthesis with generative adversarial networks. IEEE Access. 2020;8:63514–37.
49. Arora A, Arora A. Generative adversarial networks and synthetic patient data: current challenges and future perspectives. Fut Healthc J. 2022;9(2):190–3.
50. Rajagopal S, et al. Are generative AI systems capable of supporting information needs of patients? arXiv preprint arXiv. 2024:2402.00234.
51. Kovacova M, Kevicky F, Popescu GH. Generative artificial intelligence-driven healthcare systems in patient record analysis, in disease diagnosis and monitoring, and in customized treatment plans. Contemp Read Law Soc J. 2023;15(1):152.
52. Guhan P, Awasthi N, Bussell K, Manocha D, Reeves G, Bera A. Developing an effective and automated patient engagement estimator for telehealth: a machine learning approach. arXiv preprint arXiv. 2020:2011.08690.
53. Choi E, Biswal S, Malin B, Duke J, Stewart WF, Sun J. Generating multi-label discrete patient records using generative adversarial networks. In: Machine learning for healthcare conference. PMLR; 2017. p. 286–305.
54. Wang S. SeqMed: recommending medication combination with sequence generative adversarial nets. In: 2020 IEEE international conference on Bioinformatics and Biomedicine (BIBM), vol. 2020. p. 2664–71. https://doi.org/10.1109/BIBM49941.2020.9313196.
55. Singh P, Kirar JS. Integration of generative AI and deep tabular data learning architecture for heart attack prediction. In: Verma A, Verma P, Pattanaik KK, Dhurandher SK, Woungang I, editors. Advanced network technologies and intelligent computing. Cham: Springer; 2024. p. 303–17.
56. Bhagawati M, Paul S. Generative adversarial network-based deep learning framework for cardiovascular disease risk prediction. In: 2024 5th international conference on Innovative Trends in Information Technology (ICITIIT); 2024. p. 1–4. https://doi.org/10.1109/ICITIIT61487.2024.10580562.
57. Bommasani R, et al. On the opportunities and risks of foundation models. arXiv preprint arXiv. 2021:2108.07258.
58. Kaddour J, Harris J, Mozes M, Bradley H, Raileanu R, McHardy R. Challenges and applications of large language models. arXiv preprint arXiv. 2023:2307.10169.
59. Zhao WX, et al. A survey of large language models. arXiv preprint arXiv. 2023:2303.18223.
60. Chang Y, et al. A survey on evaluation of large language models. ACM Trans Intell Syst Technol. 2024;15(3):1–45.
61. Devlin J. Bert: pre-training of deep bidirectional transformers for language understanding. arXiv preprint arXiv. 2018:1810.04805.
62. Brown T, et al. Language models are few-shot learners. Adv Neural Inf Process Syst. 2020;33:1877–901.
63. Achiam J, et al. Gpt-4 technical report. arXiv preprint arXiv. 2023:2303.08774.
64. Touvron H, et al. Llama 2: open foundation and fine-tuned chat models. arXiv preprint arXiv. 2023:2307.09288.
65. Thirunavukarasu AJ, Ting DSJ, Elangovan K, Gutierrez L, Tan TF, Ting DSW. Large language models in medicine. Nat Med. 2023;29(8):1930–40.
66. Singhal K, et al. Large language models encode clinical knowledge. Nature. 2023;620(7972):172–80.
67. Rajkomar A, et al. Deciphering clinical abbreviations with a privacy protecting machine learning system. Nat Commun. 2022;13(1):7456.
68. Sezgin E, Sirrianni J, Linwood SL. Operationalizing and implementing pretrained, large artificial intelligence linguistic models in the US health care system: outlook of generative pretrained transformer 3 (GPT-3) as a service model. JMIR Med Inform. 2022;10(2):e32875.
69. Liu P, Yuan W, Fu J, Jiang Z, Hayashi H, Neubig G. Pre-train, prompt, and predict: a systematic survey of prompting methods in natural language processing. ACM Comput Surv. 2023;55(9):1–35.

70. Zhao H, et al. Explainability for large language models: a survey. ACM Trans Intell Syst Technol. 2024;15(2):1–38.
71. Wen B, Norel R, Liu J, Stappenbeck T, Zulkernine F, Chen H. Leveraging large language models for patient engagement: the power of conversational AI in digital health. arXiv preprint arXiv. 2024:2406.13659.
72. Bauer B, Norel R, Leow A, Rached ZA, Wen B, Cecchi G. Using large language models to understand suicidality in a social media–based taxonomy of mental health disorders: linguistic analysis of reddit posts. JMIR Ment Health. 2024;11:e57234.
73. Zhou H, Chen E, Wen S, Wang Y, Norel K. Large language models as a tool for cognitive stimulation: chatbot book clubs for seniors. In: IEEE international conference on digital health; 2024.
74. Hayward R. Generative artificial intelligence-driven healthcare systems in medical imaging analysis, in clinical decision support, and in patient engagement and monitoring. Contemp Read Law Soc Justice. 2023;15(1):63–80.
75. Preiksaitis C, et al. The role of large language models in transforming emergency medicine: scoping review. JMIR Med Inform. 2024;12:e53787.
76. Han G, Liu W, Huang X, Borsari B. Chain-of-interaction: Enhancing large language models for psychiatric behavior understanding by dyadic contexts. arXiv preprint arXiv. 2024:2403.13786.
77. Almazrouei E, et al. The falcon series of open language models. arXiv preprint arXiv. 2023:2311.16867.
78. Jiang AQ, et al. Mistral 7B. arXiv preprint arXiv. 2023:2310.06825.
79. Chen Y, Wang Z, Wen B, Zulkernine F. Comparative analysis of open-source language models in summarizing medical text data. arXiv preprint arXiv. 2024:2405.16295.
80. Ben Abacha A, M'rabet Y, Zhang Y, Shivade C, Langlotz C, Demner-Fushman D. Overview of the MEDIQA 2021 shared task on summarization in the medical domain. In: Proceedings of the 20th workshop on biomedical language processing; 2021. p. 74–85.
81. Ben Abacha A, Demner-Fushman D. On the summarization of consumer health questions. In: Proceedings of the 57th annual meeting of the association for computational linguistics; 2019. p. 2228–34.
82. Savery M, Ben Abacha A, Gayen S, Demner-Fushman D. Question-driven summarization of answers to consumer health questions. Sci Data. 2020;7(1):322.
83. Zeng G, et al. MedDialog: large-scale medical dialogue datasets. In: Proceedings of the 2020 conference on empirical methods in natural language processing (EMNLP); 2020. p. 9241–50.
84. Shi W, Mariano VY. Enhanced sentiment analysis of medical application using BERT and TextCNN. In: 2023 5th international conference on Machine Learning, Big Data and Business Intelligence (MLBDBI); 2023. p. 123–30. https://doi.org/10.1109/MLBDBI60823.2023.10482015.
85. Chatzimina ME, Papadaki HA, Pontikoglou C, Tsiknakis M. A comparative sentiment analysis of Greek clinical conversations using BERT, RoBERTa, GPT-2, and XLNet. Bioengineering. 2024;11(6) https://doi.org/10.3390/bioengineering11060521.
86. Osváth M, Yang Z, Kósa K. Analyzing narratives of patient experiences: a BERT topic modeling approach. Acta Polytechnica Hungarica. 2023;20:153–71. https://doi.org/10.12700/APH.20.7.2023.7.9.
87. Kopitar L, Stiglic G, Bedrac L, Bian J. Personalized meal planning in inpatient clinical dietetics using generative artificial intelligence: system description. In: 2024 IEEE 12th international conference on Healthcare Informatics (ICHI); 2024. p. 326–31. https://doi.org/10.1109/ICHI61247.2024.00049.
88. P. Mæhlum et al., "It's difficult to be neutral – human and LLM-based sentiment annotation of patient comments," 2024.
89. Dey AK. ChatGPT in diabetes care: an overview of the evolution and potential of generative artificial intelligence model like ChatGPT in augmenting clinical and patient outcomes in the management of diabetes. Int J Diabetes Technol. 2023;2(2):66–72.

90. He Y, Zhu Z, Zhang Y, Chen Q, Caverlee J. Infusing disease knowledge into BERT for health question answering. Medical Inference and Disease Name Recognition; 2020.
91. Ren F, Zhou Y. CGMVQA: a new classification and generative model for medical visual question answering. IEEE Access. 2020;8:50626–36. https://doi.org/10.1109/ACCESS.2020.2980024.
92. Turek M. Explainable artificial intelligence (XAI). Defense Advanced Research Projects Agency; 2018.
93. Selvaraj S. Empowering patients with AI-driven personalized care: the transformative power of generative AI and healthcare data integration. Int J Sci Res. 2024;13(7):337–43.
94. Hueso M, Álvarez R, Marí D, Ribas-Ripoll V, Lekadir K, Vellido A. Is generative artificial intelligence the next step toward a personalized hemodialysis? Rev Investig Clin. 2023;75(6):309–17.
95. Bird M, et al. A generative co-design framework for healthcare innovation: development and application of an end-user engagement framework. Res Involv Engagem. 2021;7:1–12.
96. Yim D, Khuntia J, Parameswaran V, Meyers A. Preliminary evidence of the use of generative AI in health care clinical services: systematic narrative review. JMIR Med Inform. 2024;12(1):e52073.
97. Jebamani BJA, Murugeswari R, Nagaraj P. Online appointment management system in hospitals using distributed resource allocation algorithm. In: Sentimental analysis and deep learning: proceedings of ICSADL 2021. Springer; 2022. p. 291–301.
98. Quevedo G. Revolutionizing patient interaction using generative AI in healthcare. [Online]. Available: https://www.infuy.com/blog/revolutionizing-patient-interaction-using-generative-ai-in-healthcare/
99. Gupta V, Singh A, Singh H, Chaudhary E. Transforming healthcare: the role of generative AI in personalized treatment recommendations. In: AI healthcare applications and security, ethical, and legal considerations. IGI Global; 2024. p. 173–89.
100. Alruwaili M, Alsayat A, Idris M, Alanazi S, Aurangzeb K. Integration and analysis of diverse healthcare data sources: a novel solution. Comput Hum Behav. 2024;157:108221.
101. Irizarry T, DeVito Dabbs A, Curran CR. Patient portals and patient engagement: a state of the science review. J Med Internet Res. 2015;17(6):e148.
102. Samala AD, Rawas S. Generative AI as virtual healthcare assistant for enhancing patient care quality. Int J Online Biomed Eng. 2024;20(5):174–87.
103. Enhancing patient engagement with GenAI. [Online]. Available: https://www.pwc.ie/industries/healthcare/publications/enhancing-patient-engagement-through-genai.html
104. Tertulino R, Antunes N, Morais H. Privacy in electronic health records: a systematic mapping study. J Public Health (Bangkok). 2024;32(3):435–54.
105. Tucker K, et al. Protecting patient privacy when sharing patient-level data from clinical trials. BMC Med Res Methodol. 2016;16:5–14.
106. Nugent C, et al. Using generative AI to assist with technology adoption assessment. In: International conference on ubiquitous computing and ambient intelligence. Springer; 2023. p. 202–7.
107. Reddy S. Generative AI in healthcare: an implementation science informed translational path on application, integration and governance. Implement Sci. 2024;19(1):27.
108. Hulsen T. Explainable artificial intelligence (XAI): concepts and challenges in healthcare. AI. 2023;4(3):652–66.
109. Ferrara E. Fairness and bias in artificial intelligence: a brief survey of sources, impacts, and mitigation strategies. Science. 2023;6(1):3.
110. Sai S, Gaur A, Sai R, Chamola V, Guizani M, Rodrigues JJPC. Generative ai for transformative healthcare: a comprehensive study of emerging models, applications, case studies and limitations. IEEE Access. 2024;12:31078–106.

Application of Generative AI in Drug Discovery

Amirfarhad Farhadi, Azadeh Zamanifar, and Miad Faezipour

1 Introduction (Table 1)

Drug discovery is a critical activity that plays a significant role in society's health. Every medicine undergoes a lengthy process and goes through clinical trials for testing and final evaluation before being distributed in the marketplace [1]. Moreover, drug discovery has some ethical limitations due to the use of animals in clinical tests and the potential risks to humans. Therefore, researchers and scholars seek out cutting-edge approaches to address these issues in the field of the pharmaceutical industry.

In recent years, drug discovery has been revolutionized by AI technology. De novo drug discovery is time-consuming, more than decade in some case and also very expensive, more than a billion dollar. According to Deep Pharma Intelligence, as of March 2023, at least 14 drugs fully generated by AI have entered clinical trials [1]. Toxicity and lack of efficacy account for greater than 60% of all drug failures [2]. The traditional approach to drug discovery is akin to a pipeline with targets, leads and molecules each needing to meet pre-set success criteria to progress towards clinical development and ultimately the market [2].

One of the approaches in computer-aided drug discovery is the use of digital twins, which are virtual models that replicate the biological and pharmacological properties of a drug, biological system, or disease state. By leveraging AI, machine

A. Farhadi (✉) · A. Zamanifar
Department of Computer Engineering, Science and Research Branch, Islamic Azad University, Tehran, Iran
e-mail: amir.farhadi@srbiau.ac.ir; azamanifar@srbiau.ac.ir

M. Faezipour
School of Engineering Technology, Purdue University, West Lafayette, IN, USA
e-mail: mfaezipo@purdue.edu

A. Zamanifar, M. Faezipour (eds.), *Application of Generative AI in Healthcare Systems*, https://doi.org/10.1007/978-3-031-82963-5_6

Table 1 Abbreviation Full Form

AI	Artificial Intelligence
GAN	Generative Adversarial Network
VAE	Variational Autoencoder
LLM	Large Language Model
RL	Reinforcement Learning
SMILE	Simplified Molecular Input Line Entry System
RNN	Recurrent Neural Network
LSTM	Long Short-Term Memory
GRU	Gated Recurrent Unit
GPU	Graphics Processing Unit
GDT	Global Distance Test
PCA	Principal Component Analysis
t-SNE	t-distributed Stochastic Neighbor Embedding
UMAP	Uniform Manifold Approximation and Projection
CNN	Convolutional Neural Network
PSO	Particle Swarm Optimization
GA	Genetic Algorithm

learning, and simulation techniques, digital twins aim to create a dynamic and data-driven representation of biological processes and disease mechanisms.

After 2012, with the introduction of deep learning and outstanding results in competitions like Kaggle, there was a significant shift in the field. The emergence of GenAI models, such as Generative Adversarial Networks (GANs) and Variational Autoencoders (VAEs), marked the first step in this transformation. This was followed by the introduction of transformer models and large language models (LLMs) like ChatGPT-3.5, Gemini, and Llama [3]. Simultaneously, advancements in hardware, GPUs, and computational processors have further accelerated these developments.

AI has had a significant impact not only on machine learning methods but also on cheminformatics and drug discovery. One of the key areas where AI has revolutionized drug discovery is through advancements in protein folding technology, which are essential for understanding molecular interactions. In 2020, DeepMind introduced AlphaFold, which revolutionized the field of protein folding by achieving an accuracy of over 90% in the Global Distance Test (GDT_TS). This outstanding result has redefined protein structure prediction methods and established a new benchmark in the field.

Nowadays, many pharmaceutical companies employ AI techniques to enhance their ability to handle large amounts of data. Specifically, many of them use in-house AI, machine learning techniques, and generative models to accelerate drug discovery and drug repurposing. For instance, predicting molecular characteristics with high precision is crucial in the drug development process. To save money on R&D, computational studies can screen and enhance predicted molecular features before costly animal and clinical testing [4]. Therefore, researchers in the fields of cheminformatics and machine learning try to leverage GenAI models to enhance efficiency and drastically decrease the cost and duration of drug discovery and drug repurposing.

Basically, generative models generate new data samples similar to the original data distribution. Early generative models, such as Gaussian Mixture Models and Hidden Markov Models, were introduced but were limited in complexity and applications. Afterward, with the introduction of deep learning and its advantages new generative models, such as Generative Adversarial Networks (GANs) were developed, where a generator and discriminator compete against each other. The GAN approach, the generator creates new molecules that are similar to the original data. The key goal of the GAN is to fool the discriminator into believing that these molecules are original. In the next step, the discriminator evaluates whether the molecules are real or fake. This iteration continues to identify original molecules that are pivotal in drug discovery [5].

GANs have shown promising results and have been a breakthrough compared to the aforementioned methods. Another generative paradigm has introduced around the same time is Variational Auto Encoder (VAE). This method leverages probabilistic approach to learn latent space representation. In general, a VAE has two parts: the encoder and the decoder. The encoder maps the input molecules to a latent space, learning the underlying distribution of the molecules. The decoder then reconstructs these molecules from the latent space. By doing so, a VAE can produce novel molecules that are similar to the original ones [6].

Employing Recurrent Neural Networks (RNN) in the context of deep neural network is very popular due to their potential to handling sequential data and capturing temporal dependencies. Some well-known RNN models are Long Short Term Memory (LSTM) and Gated Recurrent Unit (GRU). In drug discovery, RNN architectures are mainly used for sequences of atoms and Simplified Molecular Input Line Entry System (SMILES) strings. RNNs can be applied to large datasets of molecules to learn patterns and relationships between molecular components.

Another type of generative model is flow-based which learn transformation from simple distribution like Gaussian to complex distributions. These models learn transformation to map data to a latent space [7]. Leveraging graph representations due to the nature of molecular structures can be beneficial. In this approach, atoms are used as nodes of the graph, and chemical bonds as edges [8]. Two factors are crucial in graph representation: first, the molecular representation, and second, the graph-based features.

Reinforcement learning (RL) has shown significant potential for dealing with complex decision-making problems [9]. Essentially, the ability of RL to apply rewards and penalties could be beneficial for drug design in the pharmaceutical industry [7]. Training a reinforcement learning (RL) agent to generate molecules for drug discovery is one of the practical applications of RL in this field. In the section on RL in drug discovery, we elaborate further on this approach.

In recent years, Transformer-based generative models have made significant advancements in the field of GenAI. In fact these models are a type of neural network that embedded attention mechanisms, for instances ChatGPT, BERT, and Vision Transformers. In drug discovery, Transformer-based models are employed for molecule generation and optimization. For example, ChemBERTa uses a

Transformer architecture to represent chemical compounds. Additionally, these models are used to predict how different drugs interact with different type of biological targets which is crucial for both drug discovery and repurposing.

Another type of generative model is the diffusion model. One advantage of this model is its ability to generate high-quality data. This approach has three phases: in the first phase, known as the forward diffusion process, random noise is added to the samples, making them noise-like. In the second phase, the reverse diffusion process, these noise-like samples are refined and denoised. Finally, neural networks are trained to perform the reverse diffusion process. In the context of drug discovery, this involves first adding random noise to generated molecules until they become indistinguishable from random noise. In the next step, the noise is removed step by step by training classical neural networks or deep neural networks [10, 11].

In this book chapter, we discuss the application of GenAI techniques and frameworks in drug discovery and repurposing. Furthermore, we survey real-world applications of GenAI in the pharmaceutical industry. In the next section, we introduce deep learning methods in general. Following that, we cover specific GenAI models in order: GANs, VAEs, Transformer-based models, RNNs, flow-based models, and, lastly, diffusion models.

2 Generative Adversarial Network (GAN)

When generative adversarial networks (GANs) were first presented in 2014 [12], the deep learning community paid close attention [13, 14]. Generative adversarial networks are a kind of artificial intelligence algorithm designed to solve the generative modeling problem [15]. GAN consists of two deep neural networks: the generator and the discriminator. These networks engage in a zero-sum game, posing a challenge to each other. The generator's main task is to produce fake information that can deceive the discriminator. On the other hand, the discriminator focuses on distinguishing between real and fake information generated by the generator. The training process of GAN is formulated as an optimization problem in game theory, with Nash equilibrium considered as the optimal solution [16]. To minimize the loss of both the generator and the discriminator, gradient-based algorithms are employed simultaneously [14, 17].

GANs are able to generate samples from a predicted probability distribution. This network is one of the most successful generative models due to two main reasons:

1. GANs employ a unique adversarial training technique, which is a zero-sum game between the generator and the discriminator. Each module tries to outperform the other: the generator attempts to fool the discriminator by generating fake samples that resemble the original data, while the discriminator tries to distinguish between the fake samples and the real data.
2. GANs use a non-parametric method that does not rely on specific parameters like the VAE method. Instead, GANs learn directly from the target distribution.

In GAN model training sample x from unknown distribution $p_{data}(x)$. The target of GAN model that learn the $p_{model}(x)$ that approximate the $p_{data}(x)$. A simple way to approximate the $p_{data}(x)$ is to estimate function $p_{model}(x;\theta)$ regulate by parameter θ and find parameter values that resemble $p_{model}(x)$ to $p_{data}(x)$. One of the typical approaches for generative models, such as GANs, is maximum likelihood estimation (MLE), a statistical method used to estimate the parameters of a model. In this approach, minimizing the Kullback-Leibler divergence between $p_{model}(x)$ and $p_{data}(x)$ is typically employed [15].

Currently, researchers and scholars in the field of GenAI tend to favor deep neural network methods over traditional neural networks. Consequently, the capabilities of deep neural networks enable the estimation of more complex tasks and functions.

2.1 GAN in Drug Discovery

In general, deep learning models, specifically GANs, show promising performance in the field of de novo drug discovery. As shown in Fig. 1, an illustration of the GAN approach for molecule generation in drug discovery. In the context of GAN-based drug discovery and design, three main categories can be identified: molecular de novo design, dimensionality reduction of single-cell data, and, last but not least, de novo peptide design [18]. It is worth mentioning that pure GAN-based studies are still limited; however, hybrid methods incorporating techniques such as RL [19,

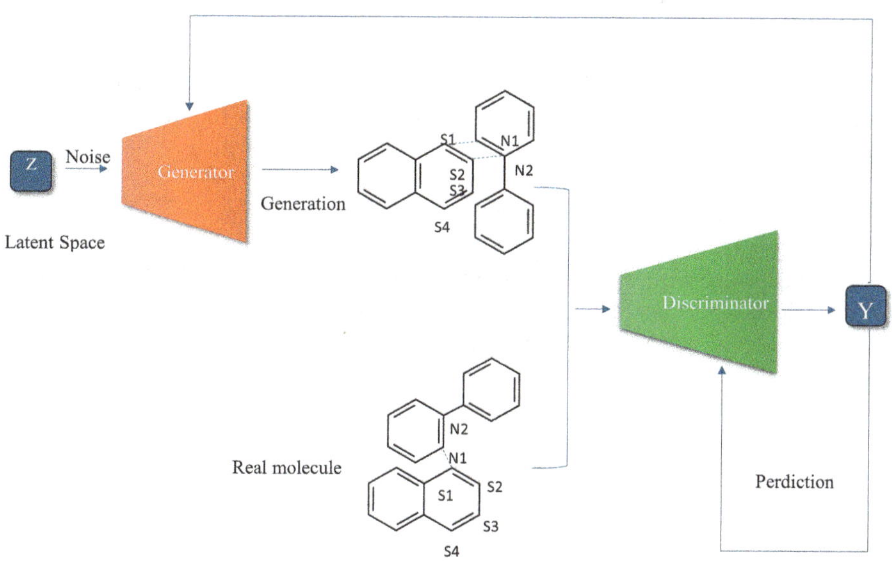

Fig. 1 Illustration of a GAN model for molecular generation

20], autoencoder [21], and other variations of GANs, like latent GAN [22], are being explored.

In molecular de novo design, how molecules are represented is essential in chemoinformatic, as it influences all the steps that follow in the analysis [23].

2.2 Molecular De Novo Design in GAN

Creating new molecules during screening and development of molecules design over the two decades [24]. Molecule representations are mainly in four forms. The first and foremost is SMILES [25] and string form; the second is based on images [26, 27], specifically 2D custom images; the third is graph-based representation [28]; and the last is tensor-based representation [29].

One of the advantages of GANs is their ability to produce continuous output values, such as vectors in images. However, since the structure of molecules is discrete, GANs face challenges in this context. To address this, previous works have combined GANs with approaches such as reinforcement learning and policy gradient methods to fine-tune the weights in the generative module, which generates de novo molecules.

Another approach that can be combined with GANs is the use of an autoencoder. In this approach, the autoencoder acts as an encoder to convert continuous data into a latent vector, which is then decoded to chemical structure by the decoder [18].

druGAN [30] is one such model that combines an autoencoder and GAN. Specifically, druGAN utilizes a generative adversarial autoencoder with certain advantages over VAE, such as adjustability in molecular fingerprints, the ability to process large datasets efficiently, and improved performance in unsupervised pretraining for regression models [30]. druGAN is capable of creating novel chemical structures that could be used in anti-cancer processes. druGAN was implemented using the PubChem [31] database, which consists of more than 70 million molecules.

2.2.1 Dimension Reduction of Single-Cell in GAN

Traditional dimension reduction techniques in machine learning, such as PCA, t-SNE, and UMAP, use classical machine learning methods. However, in recent years, deep learning methods like deep neural networks, CNNs, and GAN-based approaches have shown promising results and revolutionized these traditional methods.

Nowadays, single-cell sequencing is a cutting-edge technique in the pharmaceutical industry used to assess the performance of individual cells [32–34]. Some studies have employed GANs for dimensionality reduction in the context of drug discovery [33, 35]. Clustering GAN is a paradigm of this approach, which clusters the latent space based on GAN methods [35].

2.3 De Novo Peptide and Protein Design

The goal of de novo peptide and protein design is to create new peptides and proteins based on the physical principles of protein folding [18, 36]. Peptides are short chains of amino acids; however, proteins are macromolecules that consist of amino acids [36].

3 VAE

A Variational Autoencoder (VAE) is a type of GenAI that learns a latent representation of data and generates new data similar to the input [37]. A VAE consists of two parts: an encoder, which maps the input to a latent space and provides a probabilistic representation, and a decoder, which reconstructs the input from the latent space [38]. As shown in Fig. 2, the general schematic of the VAE architecture in the context of drug discovery is based on an encoder and a decoder module to learn latent space representation.

3.1 Applications of VAE in Drug Discovery

1. One of the challenging tasks in drug discovery using GenAI is that molecules are often represented in a discrete format, such as SMILES strings. However, converting discrete data to continuous data is challenging. Since a continuous latent space is more flexible than a discrete one, VAEs can encode molecular data into a continuous latent space for this purpose. Specifically, this approach enables interpolation between molecules and the generation of new compounds.
2. VAE can generate new molecules by sampling from the learned latent space. This leads to the generation of novel compounds. As this latent space is continuous, it allows for smooth transitions, which are crucial for exploring previously uncharted regions.

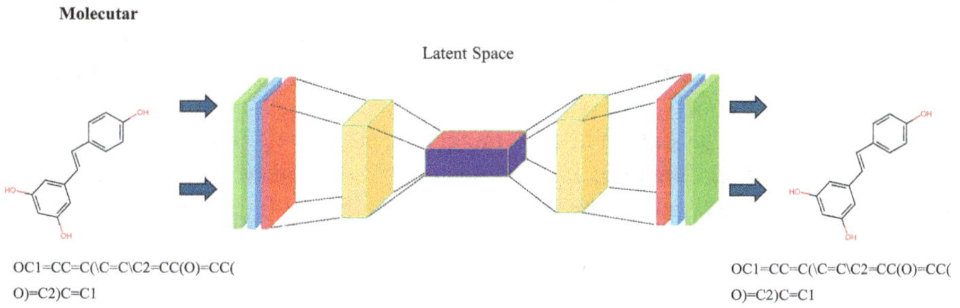

Fig. 2 Framework of a VAE for molecules generation

3. Property prediction is one of the crucial applications of VAE in drug discovery. VAE can be conditioned to optimize specific properties during the generation process.

4 RL in Drug Discovery

RL is a branch of Artificial Intelligence (AI) where an agent (or agents) interacts with an environment and receives feedback in the form of rewards or penalties based on its actions [39]. Reinforcement learning is the most popular technique for molecule generation [40]. As we mentioned in the introduction section, RL is one of the preferred approaches in drug discovery, particularly in its pure form or in combination with other approaches.

We can categorize RL in drug discovery into four categories as follow:

4.1 *De Novo Drug Design in RL*

The aim of **de novo** design is to create new molecules from scratch using reinforcement learning (RL) techniques. Atance et al. [41] aim to leverage a graph-based deep generative model, specifically using RL to fine-tune the generative models with a desired set of properties. Another study [40] in this context is to leverage GPT agents for drug generation. Exploring molecular structures using Large Language Models (LLMs) and pre-trained models offers several advantages, such as speeding up the preclinical phase and generally reducing the time and cost of drug discovery. One application of reinforcement learning in LLMs involves interaction with humans, known as Reinforcement Learning from Human Feedback (RLHF). In fact, RLHF leverages human input to guide the model toward more desirable results.

As shown in Fig. 3, the RL architecture in drug repurposing is based on the actor-critic model, which is a popular approach in RL that combines policy-based and value-based methods.

The pivotal issue in molecular generation for formulation is the scoring function $s(x)$, which evaluates molecular properties. $s(x)$ also called as oracle due to estimate of the variable x, and the $s(x)$ is the real number [40]. In Eq. (1), the scoring function ranges from zero to one.

Values closer to one indicate better molecular properties. In Eq. (1), $t(x)$ represents the transformer function, $p(x)$ is molecules probability predictor, and w_i is weighted used in the combination of the oracle and then optimize Eq. (1).

$$s(x) = t(p(x)) or\, s(x) = \sum w_i t_i (p_i(x)), \sum w_i = 1 \tag{1}$$

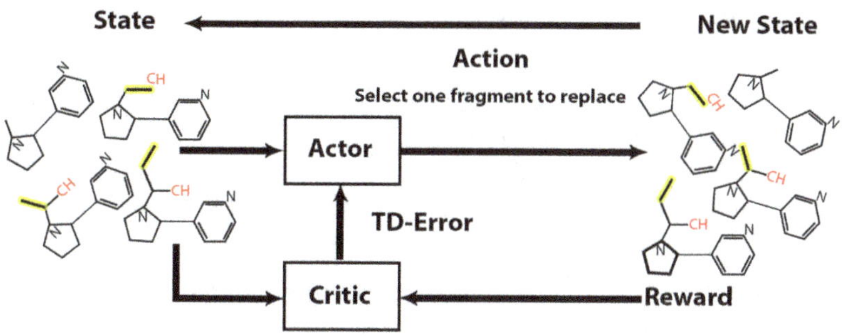

Fig. 3 Illustration of Actor-Critic RL in Molecular Generation

In general, studies focus on the final set of generated molecule candidates, thereby bypassing computational and time costs.

4.2 *Molecular Docking Optimization in RL*

Molecular docking is a key computational method used to analyze how small molecules (such as ligands) interact with target proteins (receptors) [42, 43]. Optimization in molecular docking plays a significant role in improving the accuracy of predictions and enabling more reliable drug candidate identification. In 2019, N. Stahl et al. proposed a fragment-based reinforcement learning approach using an actor-critic model for the generation of new molecules with optimal properties [44] in this method [44] both the actor and critic use LSTM. More specifically, after initiating the set of lead molecules, the fragments are replaced by a balanced binary tree.

$$v^{\pi}(\mathrm{s}) = E^{\pi}\left[r_{t+1} + \gamma r_{t+2} + \gamma_2 r_{t+3} + \ldots | s_t = \mathrm{s}\right] \tag{2}$$

$$= E^{\pi}\left[r_{t+1} + \gamma\, v^{\pi}\left(s_{t+1}\right) | s_t = \mathrm{s}\right] \tag{3}$$

In Eq. (2) v^{π} (s) represents state value function, r_{t+1} represents reward in t + 1 time step and E^{π} is expected value in policy π. To modify molecules, they must be in a format that can be easily adjusted. For this purpose, a binary structure is desirable. Afterward, the molecules are divided into fragments, and based on the actor-critic method, the model identifies which fragments should remain and which ones must be replaced.

4.3 *Drug Repurposing in RL*

Drug repurposing, also called drug repositioning, is the discovery of new therapeutic uses for existing or previously developed drugs. The advantage of drug repurposing is that it reduces the cost of drug discovery compared to developing new drugs from scratch [45]. In the context of drug repurposing, the state, action, and reward fundamental elements of RL are defined as follows:

- **State**: The environment, which may include information about biological factors, diseases, and molecular data.
- **Action**: The decisions made by the RL agent, such as selecting molecules for interaction.
- **Reward**: The reward is a pivotal aspect of RL. Rewards can vary, such as the effectiveness of the drug in treatment, its side effects, or the clinical evaluation of the drug.

Stork et al. [46] proposed a method that leverages a graph traversal algorithm. In reinforcement learning (RL), multi-agent methods involve multiple agents interacting with each other in a shared environment. Each agent interacts with both the environment and other agents to maximize its reward. Leveraging multi-agent RL could be beneficial for drug repurposing. Due to the complexity of biological datasets and the intricate interactions within them, multi-agent RL can address these challenges by coordinating the actions of multiple agents. One promising approach is to explore the drug-disease space, where each agent represents a specific method or approach for modeling drug-disease interactions.

5 RNN in Drug Discovery

Recurrent neural networks are a class neural networks that are applied in sequential data. In recent years generative RNN models are applies vastly in different due to cope sequential data. The contribution of the RNN in drug discovery is as follow:

1. **Molecules Representation**: one of the applications of drug discovery in RNN is molecules representation SMILES strings, that are sequential structure in this way, LSTM and GRU are common methods that used.
2. **De Novo Drug Design**: In de novo drug design, generative RNNs are employed to handle sequential data. The RNN is trained on a large dataset of known molecules, which are typically represented as molecular graphs or SMILES strings. To ensure proper generalization, the training dataset should include a wide range of drug-like molecules.

Examples of de novo drug design in drug discovery can be divided into two main categories. The first is polyketide synthesis, where an RNN model has been used to generate new polyketide structures. The second is the development of antibiotics that inhibit bacterial activity while minimizing side effects.

5.1 Long Short-Term Memory (LSTM)

LSTM was introduced by Hochreiter and Schmid Huber in 1997 [47]. LSTM is a type of RNN designed to address the vanishing gradient problem: during weight updates, gradients become too small, making it difficult for the network to adjust the weights properly. To handle this issue, LSTM employs gating mechanisms specifically, input gates, output gates, and forget gates. These gates allow the network to maintain and update information during sequences of data. Furthermore, LSTM captures long-term dependencies in sequential data [48]. As a result, LSTMs have wide applicability in different applications such as NLP, speech recognition, and drug discovery [49, 50].

LSTMs have been employed in GenAI for drug discovery, specifically for de novo design. Training an LSTM on a large dataset of molecular structures represented as SMILES strings aims to learn the syntax and patterns of chemical representations. After training, the LSTM can generate new SMILES for potential candidate molecule structures. This approach allows for the exploration of chemical space and the generation of compounds with desired properties by combining it with reinforcement learning techniques.

5.2 Gated Recurrent Unit (GRU)

A Gated Recurrent Unit (GRU) is a type of RNN introduced in 2014 by Kyunghyun Cho and colleagues [51]. GRUs are used to maintain dependencies in sequential data such as natural language processing, speech recognition, and drug discovery [52].

GRU has two gated:

Reset gate (r_t): decide how to combine new input with previous memory
Update gate (z_t): determines how much the past information retain

Compared to LSTMs, GRUs have a simpler architecture and fewer parameters, which can reduce the computational cost [53].

Application of GRU in drug discovery could categorize as follow:

Molecules representation: molecules are usually representing text-based structure as SMILES
Model training: GRU model has the ability to train on large dataset of SMILES
Molecules generation: afterward training, new character SMILES predict and molecules generate by GRU.

Properties optimization: after molecules generation with some algorithm such as Genetic Algorithm (GA), Particle Swarm Optimization (PSO), or with RL technique models can guided to generate molecules with specific properties (e.g., less side effect or low toxicity) ability of GRU to combine with another generative models such as VAE and GAN cause more capability of more generatively [54, 55]. For instance, combining with VAE allow to encoded more molecules properties to latent space or with GAN model allow more diversity and fidelity of generated data [56]. Furthermore, using some techniques such as transfer learning allow model to leveraging previous knowledge from pre-trained models. In this approach in simple way freeze some layer of CNN and modify the last layers of networks [57].

6 Transformer-Based Drug Discovery

Transformers are a neural network architecture introduced by Vaswani et al. in 2017 [58]. One of the key innovations of Transformers is the use of the self-attention mechanism. The self-attention mechanism allows models to weigh different parts of the input sequence when generating representations [59, 60]. Furthermore, the self-attention mechanism can capture long-range dependencies more effectively than traditional RNNs, which rely on sequential processing and can struggle with such dependencies. Another advantage of self-attention is that it enables models to process data in parallel, speeding up computation [61]. As shown in Fig. 4, the architecture of the transformer processes the input sequence representing the chemical structure. The multi-head attention and positional encoding layers capture relationships between the features.

6.1 *Applications of Transformer in Drug Discovery*

1. **Molecular Representation Learning**: Molecules can be represented using SMILES strings or graph representations—where atoms are nodes and bonds are edges. Employing Transformers has the advantage of learning richer representations of molecular structures.
2. **Molecule Generation**: Transformers are able to generate molecules by predicting the next token in SMILES strings or constructing graph structures.
3. **Property Prediction**: Transformers can learn to predict molecular properties such as toxicity and binding affinity by training on datasets.
4. **Reaction Prediction**: Transformers can predict the outcomes of chemical reactions, sometimes in combination with reinforcement learning.

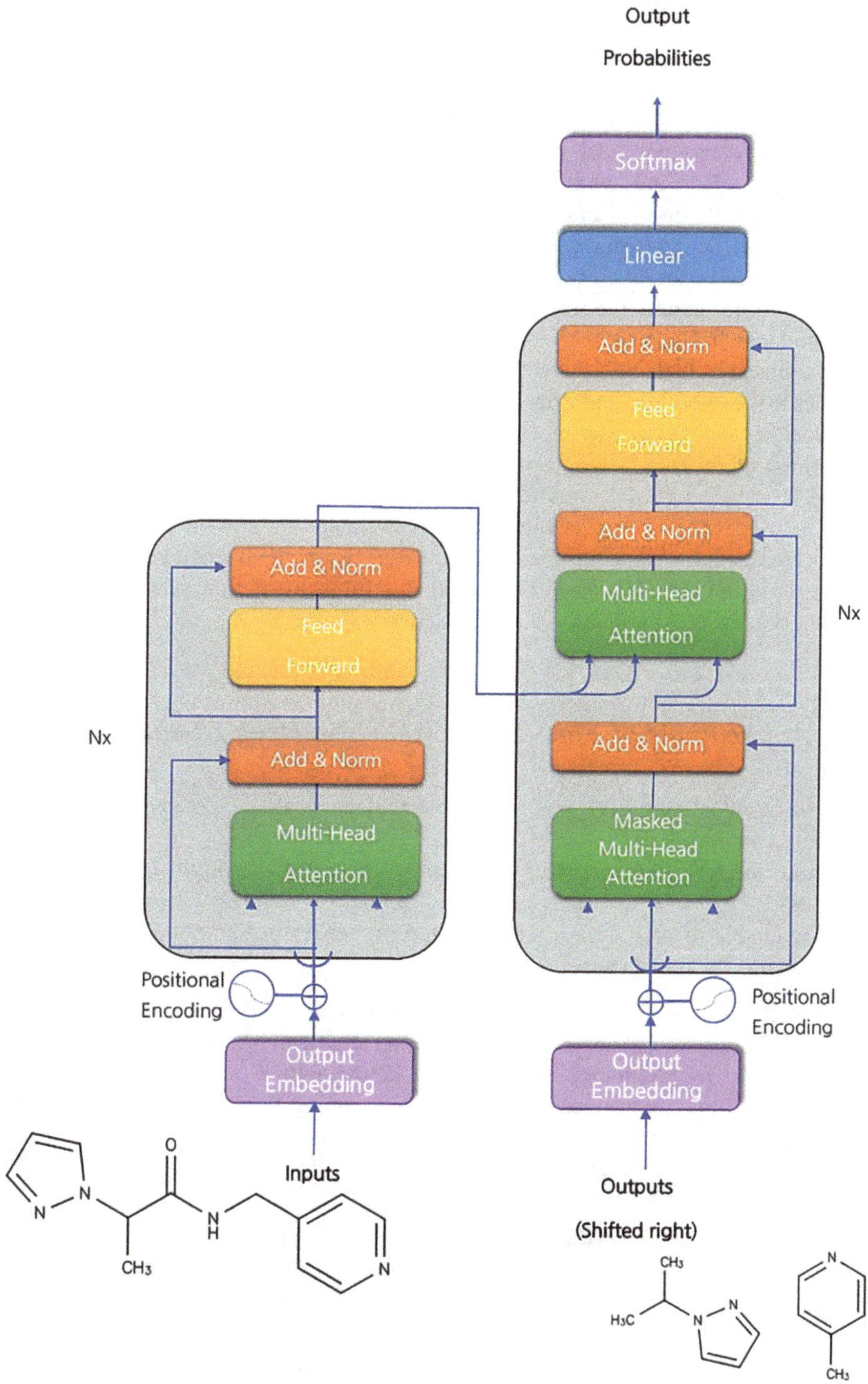

Fig. 4 Schematic of a transformer-based framework for drug discovery

7 Flow-Based Models

Flow-based models are a type of GenAI that transform simple probability distributions into complex ones by employing invertible and differentiable mappings [62] precisely, flow-based model is series of invertible transformation for mapping between data space and latent space. Unlike GANs and VAEs, flow-based models estimate exact likelihoods and allow for tractable inference [63]. Due to the invertible nature of their transformations, flow-based models enable efficient sampling from the model. Moreover, flow-based models have more stable training in comparison to other generative models like GANs, which can suffer from issues like mode collapse [64].

Flow-based models also have applications in image generation, anomaly detection, density estimation, and drug discovery [65]. Flow-based models impact drug discovery by generating new molecules with desired properties and facilitating the exploration of chemical space [66, 67].

The flow-based model aims to learn a sequence of invertible transformations $f_\theta = f_L \circ ... \circ f_1$ between complex high-dimensional data $x \sim p_x(X)$ and $Z \sim p_Z(Z)$ in a latent space with the same number of dimensions where the latent distribution $p_Z(Z)$ is easy to model [68]. Figure 5 illustrate the architecture of flow-based model that commonly used in computational drug discovery.

7.1 Applications of Flow-Based Models in Drug Discovery

1. Flow-based models can generate novel molecules that meet specific criteria, such as solubility.
2. These models can optimize molecular properties through gradient-based methods.
3. They enable inverse design with targeted properties by sampling from specific regions of the latent space.

- Zhang and Wang in 2020 [68] proposed method based on flow-based model that employed Graph Neural network structure. This approach has two steps, in step one learning latent representation and step two, generation of molecules in the graph structure. MoFlow allows model to invertible mapping from molecules graph and latent representation.

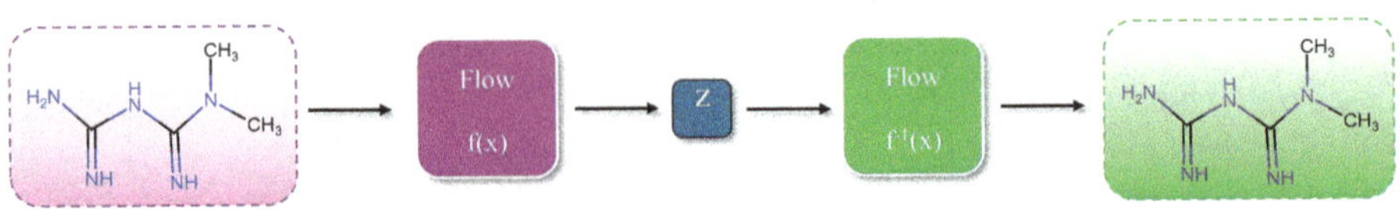

Fig. 5 Overview of flow-based model approach molecular generation

8 Diffusion Models

Diffusion models are a type of generative model that outperform in generating high-quality synthetic data compared to other generative models such as GANs and VAEs [10, 69]. Figure 6 shows a diffusion-based model used for generating new molecular structures in drug discovery. The model gradually changes a molecule step by step, as shown by the sequence of molecules with slight differences. Starting from a known molecule (left), small amounts of noise are added or removed until it reaches a simplified representation, called latent space Z (right). This process can be reversed to generate new, valid molecular structures. By exploring different steps, the model helps researchers design new molecules with specific properties for tasks such as drug design and optimization.

The diffusion process is divided into two phases:

1. **Noising**: This step starts with real data and gradually adds noise (e.g., Gaussian noise) over time steps. The noising process is typically modeled as a Markov chain, where each state depends only on the previous step.
2. **Denoising**: In this phase, the noising process is reversed, and noise is removed step by step until the original distribution is reached. Deep neural networks are leveraged to learn the parameters in this approach.

8.1 *Applications of Diffusion Models in Drug Discovery*

1. Diffusion models are employed for the generation of novel molecules by learning the underlying distribution of original molecular structures.
2. In the diffusion process, conditioning on specific molecular features can optimize them to meet ideal criteria, such as solubility and toxicity.
3. The diffusion approach can be designed to generate 3D structures, which is crucial for structure-based drug design.
4. Augmenting existing datasets by generating novel and diverse data can enhance the overall dataset.

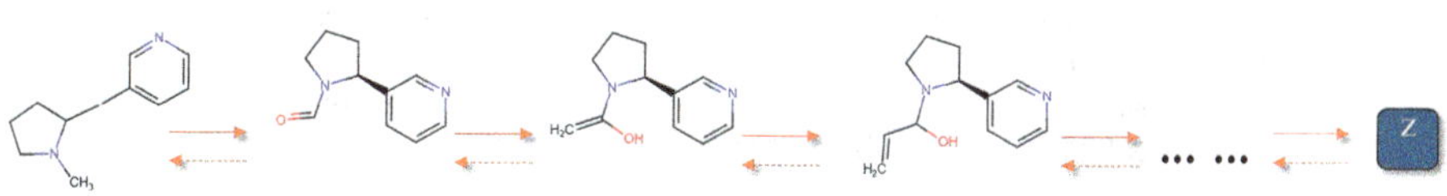

Fig. 6 Schematic of Diffusion model in drug discovery

9 Discussion

Generative AI models have become pivotal in drug discovery, each offering unique advantages and challenges. In Table 2, we provide a detailed comparison of the most prominent generative models used in this field, including GANs, VAEs, LSTMs, GRUs, flow-based models, diffusion models, transformer-based models, and RL-based models. These models differ in their ability to handle chemical

Table 2 Comparison between generative models in drug discovery

Method	Advantage	Disadvantage
GAN	Generates novel drug-like molecules with realistic chemical properties. Can learn directly from molecular data without handcrafting features.	Training instability (mode collapse) can lead to poor chemical diversity. Hard to optimize for specific drug properties (e.g., solubility).
VAE	Useful for exploring chemical space efficiently. Captures continuous latent spaces, making drug optimization easier.	Lower quality of generated molecules compared to other models. Reconstructions may lack important chemical validity.
LSTM	Good at generating molecular sequences, particularly SMILES strings. Can handle sequential data for predicting drug properties.	Struggles with chemical validity when generating new molecules. Slow to train on large molecular datasets.
GRU	Faster training than LSTM for generating molecular sequences. Works well for small to medium-sized molecular datasets.	May not capture the full complexity of large chemical spaces. Similar challenges in chemical validity as LSTM.
Flow-based model	Generates molecules with exact likelihoods, providing more control over properties. Easier to manipulate for inverse drug design.	Computationally expensive for large molecules. Less robust in capturing all chemical variations compared to other methods.
Diffusion model	Excellent at handling large chemical datasets (e.g., molecular graphs, SMILES strings). Scalable and adaptable to various tasks like property prediction and molecular generation.	Slow generation process, making it impractical for high-throughput drug discovery pipelines. Training can be computationally expensive.
Transformer-based model	Excellent at handling large chemical datasets (e.g., molecular graphs, SMILES strings). Scalable and adaptable to various tasks like property prediction and molecular generation.	Requires significant computational resources. Risk of overfitting, especially with limited drug-related data.
RL based model	Allows objective-driven optimization (e.g., optimizing molecular efficacy, toxicity, or binding affinity). Flexible integration with other models to achieve task-specific goals.	Designing the right reward functions is complex and critical. Training is slow and computationally demanding, especially for multi-objective optimization.

complexity, scalability, and computational efficiency, offering diverse approaches depending on the specific requirements of the drug discovery pipeline. Understanding these strengths and challenges allow for informed choices when integrating AI models into pharmaceutical research.

10 Conclusion and Future Perspective

Currently, the role of GenAI in drug discovery is prominent. In this approach for facilitate the process of drug discovery or drug repurposing in one side and cost of discovery of new drug in another side cause use of generative models are crucial. Using of adversarial learning (e.g., GAN) which, have two main modules generator and discriminator which compete with each other in game-like way or VAE base on two parts decoder and encoder to learn latent space.

Advanced models to learn and generate novel molecules for sake of drug discovery for instance RNN architecture which is consist of recurrent structure such as LSTM and GRU are famous models in recurrent approach in this chapter discuss different type of generative models that employed in field of drug discovery.

Different structure of molecules like SMILES or Graph in continuous or discrete data structure have been used in GenAI model. Leveraging RL for the interactive in the molecule's generation environment based on rewards and penalties. Moreover, combination of RL with generative model in AI such as RNN or GAN architecture in de novo drug design, molecule generation, predictive modeling and optimization for drug property are applicable in this context.

In recent years Transformer-based models such as Chat gpt, Gemini, etc that based on self-attention mechanism. The future works in this era will be based on pre-trained and post-trained models in the LLM context. Furthermore, using of LLM agents that customize to handle some challenging tasks such as reasoning and autonomous behaviors.

References

1. Bordukova M, et al. Generative artificial intelligence empowers digital twins in drug discovery and clinical trials. Expert Opin Drug Discov. 2024;19(1):33–42.
2. Subramanian K. Digital twin for drug discovery and development—the virtual liver. J Indian Inst Sci. 2020;100(4):653–62.
3. Farhadi A, et al. Leveraging blockchain and ANFIS for optimal supply chain management. 2024. arXiv:2408.17161. https://doi.org/10.48550/arXiv.2408.17161.
4. Garg P, Takyar A, Bhardwaj AK. Generative artificial intelligence in drug discovery. Int J Enhanced Res Sci Technol Eng. 2024;13(4):1–9.
5. Rathod V, et al. Unlocking new possibilities in drug discovery: a GAN-based approach. In: Artificial intelligence-based healthcare systems. Cham: Springer; 2023. p. 135–44.
6. Martinelli DD. Generative machine learning for de novo drug discovery: a systematic review. Comput Biol Med. 2022;145:105403.

7. Popova M, Isayev O, Tropsha A. Deep reinforcement learning for de novo drug design. Sci Adv. 2018;4(7):eaap7885.
8. Frey NC, Gadepally V, Ramsundar B. Fastflows: flow-based models for molecular graph generation. arXiv preprint arXiv:2201.12419. 2022.
9. Farhadi A, et al. Domain adaptation in reinforcement learning: a comprehensive and systematic study. J Zhejiang Univ Sci C. 2024;25:1446–65. https://doi.org/10.1093/comjnl/bxad104
10. Xu M, et al. Geodiff: a geometric diffusion model for molecular conformation generation. arXiv preprint arXiv:2203.02923. 2022.
11. Levy D, Rector-Brooks J. Molecular fragment-based diffusion model for drug discovery. In: ICLR 2023-machine learning for drug discovery workshop. Kigali Convention Centre in Kigali, Rwanda: https://openreview.net/; 2023.
12. Goodfellow I, et al. Generative adversarial nets. Adv Neural Inf Process Syst. 2014;27.
13. Goodfellow I, Pouget-Abadie J, Mirza M, Xu B, Warde-Farley D, Ozair S, Courville A, Bengio Y. Generative adversarial nets. In: 27th advances in neural information processing systems; Montréal, Canada: NIPS Foundation; 2014.
14. Mahalegi HSM, et al. Generative adversarial networks for heterogeneous unsupervised domain adaptation detection. In: 2024 IEEE 28th international conference on intelligent engineering systems (INES). IEEE; 2024.
15. Goodfellow I, et al. Generative adversarial networks. Commun ACM. 2020;63(11):139–44.
16. Farhadi A, et al. Unsupervised domain adaptation for image classification based on deep neural networks. Intell Multimed Process Commun Syst (IMPCS). 2023;4(1):27–37.
17. Farhadi A, Sharifi A. Leveraging meta-learning to improve unsupervised domain adaptation. Comput J. 2024;67(5):1838–50.
18. Lin E, Lin C-H, Lane H-Y. Relevant applications of generative adversarial networks in drug design and discovery: molecular de novo design, dimensionality reduction, and de novo peptide and protein design. Molecules. 2020;25(14):3250.
19. Padalkar GR, et al. Drug discovery using generative adversarial network with reinforcement learning. In: 2021 international conference on computer communication and informatics (ICCCI). IEEE; 2021.
20. Tang H, et al. EarlGAN: an enhanced actor–critic reinforcement learning agent-driven GAN for de novo drug design. Pattern Recogn Lett. 2023;175:45–51.
21. Abbasi M, et al. Designing optimized drug candidates with Generative Adversarial Network. J Chem. 2022;14(1):40.
22. Prykhodko O, et al. A de novo molecular generation method using latent vector based generative adversarial network. J Chem. 2019;11:1–13.
23. Martinez-Mayorga K, et al. The impact of chemoinformatics on drug discovery in the pharmaceutical industry. Expert Opin Drug Discov. 2020;15(3):293–306.
24. Hessler G, Baringhaus K-H. Artificial intelligence in drug design. Molecules. 2018;23(10):2520.
25. Weininger D. SMILES, a chemical language and information system. 1. Introduction to methodology and encoding rules. J Chem Inf Comput Sci. 1988;28(1):31–6.
26. Goh GB, et al. Chemception: a deep neural network with minimal chemistry knowledge matches the performance of expert-developed QSAR/QSPR models. arXiv preprint arXiv:1706.06689. 2017.
27. Bjerrum EJ, Sattarov B. Improving chemical autoencoder latent space and molecular de novo generation diversity with heteroencoders. Biomol Ther. 2018;8(4):131.
28. You J, et al. Graph convolutional policy network for goal-directed molecular graph generation. Adv Neural Inf Proces Syst. 2018;31.
29. Simonovsky M, Komodakis N. Graphvae: towards generation of small graphs using variational autoencoders. In: Artificial neural networks and machine learning–ICANN 2018: 27th international conference on artificial neural networks, Rhodes, Greece, October 4–7, 2018, proceedings, part I 27. Cham: Springer; 2018.

30. Kadurin A, et al. druGAN: an advanced generative adversarial autoencoder model for de novo generation of new molecules with desired molecular properties in silico. Mol Pharm. 2017;14(9):3098–104.
31. Kim S, et al. PubChem substance and compound databases. Nucleic Acids Res. 2016;44(D1):D1202–13.
32. Vamathevan J, et al. Applications of machine learning in drug discovery and development. Nat Rev Drug Discov. 2019;18(6):463–77.
33. Lin E, Mukherjee S, Kannan S. A deep adversarial variational autoencoder model for dimensionality reduction in single-cell RNA sequencing analysis. BMC Bioinformatics. 2020;21:1–11.
34. Zeisel A, et al. Cell types in the mouse cortex and hippocampus revealed by single-cell RNA-seq. Science. 2015;347(6226):1138–42.
35. Mukherjee S, et al. Clustergan: latent space clustering in generative adversarial networks. In: Proceedings of the AAAI conference on artificial intelligence. AAAI Press; 2019. https://doi.org/10.1609/aaai.v33i01.33014610.
36. Huang P-S, Boyken SE, Baker D. The coming of age of de novo protein design. Nature. 2016;537(7620):320–7.
37. Kusner MJ, Paige B, Hernández-Lobato JM. Grammar variational autoencoder. In: International conference on machine learning. PMLR; 2017.
38. Kutsal M, Ucar F, Kati N. Computational drug discovery on human immunodeficiency virus with a customized long short-term memory variational autoencoder deep-learning architecture. CPT Pharmacometrics Syst Pharmacol. 2024;13(2):308–16.
39. Sutton RS. Reinforcement learning: an introduction. Cambridge: A Bradford Book; 2018.
40. Hu X, et al. De novo drug design using reinforcement learning with multiple gpt agents. Adv Neural Inf Proces Syst. 2024;36.
41. Atance SR, et al. De novo drug design using reinforcement learning with graph-based deep generative models. J Chem Inf Model. 2022;62(20):4863–72.
42. Jeon W, Kim D. Autonomous molecule generation using reinforcement learning and docking to develop potential novel inhibitors. Sci Rep. 2020;10(1):22104.
43. Goel M, et al. MoleGuLAR: molecule generation using reinforcement learning with alternating rewards. J Chem Inf Model. 2021;61(12):5815–26.
44. Ståhl N, et al. Deep reinforcement learning for multiparameter optimization in de novo drug design. J Chem Inf Model. 2019;59(7):3166–76.
45. Nguyen TM, et al. Counterfactual explanation with multi-agent reinforcement learning for drug target prediction. arXiv preprint arXiv:2103.12983. 2021.
46. Stork L, et al. Explainable drug repurposing in context via deep reinforcement learning. In: European semantic web conference. Springer; 2023.
47. Hochreiter S. Long short-term memory. Neural Comput. 1997;9(8):1735–80. MIT-Press.
48. Sutskever I. Sequence to sequence learning with neural networks. arXiv preprint arXiv:1409.3215. 2014.
49. Graves A, Mohamed A-r, Hinton G. Speech recognition with deep recurrent neural networks. In: 2013 IEEE international conference on acoustics, speech and signal processing. IEEE; 2013.
50. Qin Y, et al. A dual-stage attention-based recurrent neural network for time series prediction. arXiv preprint arXiv:1704.02971. 2017.
51. Cho K. Learning phrase representations using RNN encoder-decoder for statistical machine translation. arXiv preprint arXiv:1406.1078. 2014.
52. Chung J, et al. Empirical evaluation of gated recurrent neural networks on sequence modeling. arXiv preprint arXiv:1412.3555. 2014.
53. Jozefowicz R, Zaremba W, Sutskever I. An empirical exploration of recurrent network architectures. In: International conference on machine learning. PMLR; 2015.
54. Wang M, et al. Deep learning approaches for de novo drug design: an overview. Curr Opin Struct Biol. 2022;72:135–44.

55. Hung CL, Chen CC. Computational approaches for drug discovery. Drug Dev Res. 2014;75(6):412–8.
56. Olivecrona M, et al. Molecular de-novo design through deep reinforcement learning. J Chem. 2017;9:1–14.
57. Cai C, et al. Transfer learning for drug discovery. J Med Chem. 2020;63(16):8683–94.
58. Vaswani A. Attention is all you need. Adv Neural Inf Proces Syst. 2017. Long Beach, USA: 31st Conference on Neural Information Processing Systems (NIPS 2017).
59. Honda S, Shi S, Ueda HR. Smiles transformer: pre-trained molecular fingerprint for low data drug discovery. arXiv preprint arXiv:1911.04738. 2019.
60. Grechishnikova D. Transformer neural network for protein-specific de novo drug generation as a machine translation problem. Sci Rep. 2021;11(1):321.
61. Mao J, et al. Transformer-based molecular generative model for antiviral drug design. J Chem Inf Model. 2023;64(7):2733–45.
62. Rezende D, Mohamed S. Variational inference with normalizing flows. In: International conference on machine learning. PMLR; 2015.
63. Dinh L, Sohl-Dickstein J, Bengio S. Density estimation using real nvp. arXiv preprint arXiv:1605.08803. 2016.
64. Kingma DP, Dhariwal P. Glow: generative flow with invertible 1x1 convolutions. Adv Neural Inf Proces Syst. 2018;31.
65. Shi C, et al. Graphaf: a flow-based autoregressive model for molecular graph generation. arXiv preprint arXiv:2001.09382. 2020.
66. Liu J, et al. Graph normalizing flows. Adv Neural Inf Proces Syst. 2019;32.
67. Papamakarios G, Pavlakou T, Murray I. Masked autoregressive flow for density estimation. Adv Neural Inf Proces Syst. 2017;30.
68. Zang C, Wang F. Moflow: an invertible flow model for generating molecular graphs. In: Proceedings of the 26th ACM SIGKDD international conference on knowledge discovery & data mining. New York: Association for Computing Machinery; 2020.
69. Cockburn IM, Henderson R, Stern S. The diffusion of science-driven drug discovery: organizational change in pharmaceutical research. Cambridge: National Bureau of Economic Research; 1999.

Application of Generative AI in Resource Optimization in Healthcare Systems

Homayoun Safarpour Motealegh Mahalegi, Amirfarhad Farhadi, Gergő Balogh, and Eniko Nagy

1 Introduction

1.1 Background and Context

After the COVID-19 epidemic, we were all sharply reminded of how easily our planet may be susceptible to unanticipated health disasters. It was a worldwide event that shook our healthcare systems to their foundation, affecting everything from resources to healthcare delivery. This was not merely another epidemic involving many of our loved ones and acquaintances. It demonstrated that even if we have experienced significant outbreaks, including various strains of influenza and even the plague, a fresh tragedy can always strike, and sometimes we are not as prepared as we would like. At this point, a pressing question remains: Which worldwide healthcare systems handled this crisis with superior performance? Frequently, the

H. S. M. Mahalegi (✉)
Department of Software Engineering, Science and Research Branch, University of Szeged, Szeged, Hungary
e-mail: safarpour@inf.u-szeged.hu

A. Farhadi
Department of Computer Engineering, Science and Research Branch, Islamic Azad University, Tehran, Iran
e-mail: amir.farhadi@srbiau.ac.ir

G. Balogh
Department of Software Engineering, University of Szeged, Szeged, Hungary
e-mail: geryxyz@inf.u-szeged.hu

E. Nagy
Antal Bejczy Center for Intelligent Robotics, John von Neumann Faculty of Informatics, Óbuda University, Budapest, Hungary
e-mail: nagy.eniko@nik.uni-obuda.hu

A. Zamanifar, M. Faezipour (eds.), *Application of Generative AI in Healthcare Systems*, https://doi.org/10.1007/978-3-031-82963-5_7

answer lies in empowering responsible individuals who possess the capability to make decisions more efficiently, manage healthcare resources with greater precision, and provide services to patients either in person or via remote means.

Navigating the healthcare terrain nowadays is like guiding a ship over both calm and turbulent waves. There are times of innovation and development as well as ongoing difficulties needing careful planning and management. Understanding the broader context of healthcare systems highlights the critical importance of efficient resource management. Whether ensuring hospitals operate smoothly or that patients receive the best possible treatment, effective resource handling is vital for the overall success of the system. The provision of treatment is a delicate balancing act due to the high level of complexity that exists within healthcare systems. These systems intertwine the needs of patients with a multitude of challenges. A comprehensive network of physicians, nurses, technicians, and administrators, ranging from small clinics to large hospitals, collaborates to accomplish this objective. Nonetheless, despite these initiatives, the system persists under constant pressure to achieve improved outcomes with reduced resources, meet increasing demand, and curtail expenditures. Public healthcare resources in both affluent and impoverished nations are inadequate to meet demand.

1.2 Global Trends in Health and Life Expectancy

Human health has improved over the past five decades. In 1950, the worldwide average life expectancy was 46 years. By 1980, human longevity had increased to 61 years; by 1998, it had ascended to 67 years. These successes primarily originated from low- and middle-income countries and resulted from improvements in diet, sanitation, medical advancements, and enhanced public health infrastructure [1].

However, not all nations have recently experienced a rise in life expectancy. Men's life expectancy significantly decreased from 70 years in 1986 to 64 years in 1994 in the countries of the former Soviet Union. Factors contributing to this decline include elevated rates of nicotine and alcohol consumption, inadequate nutrition, depression, deterioration of the healthcare system, and economic and social instability.

Life expectancy has been drastically reduced in several African countries due to the spread of HIV/AIDS. The life expectancy is below 40 years and is declining in seven African nations. Thirteen million individuals around the globe succumb to infectious illnesses every year [2]. The death toll from AIDS was 2.8 million in 1999. The rise in international travel has allowed infectious illnesses formerly limited to certain areas to spread across national boundaries. In developed countries, noncommunicable diseases like diabetes, heart disease, cancer, and stroke are the primary causes of death. It is anticipated that in 20 years, these diseases will claim 70% of lives in low-income countries, an increase from the current 50%. In high-income countries, obesity is increasingly emerging as a significant health issue. Nevertheless, malnutrition remains an issue in low-income countries. The consumption of drugs, alcohol, and tobacco is detrimental to global health. Tobacco use is expected by 2030 to cause over 11.5 million premature deaths, mostly in low- and middle-income countries. More than 2 million individuals succumb to premature death due to food and water contamination in low- and middle-income nations. In certain regions, arsenic, lead, and silica pose health risks. Chemical and synthetic biological weapons pose a threat to public health [3].

1.3 *Significance of Resource Optimization in Healthcare*

Medical infrastructure is basic resources are important for improving healthcare outcomes across all providers, lowering costs, and making operations run more smoothly. These resources could even save patients' lives by making healthcare environments more efficient, especially when it comes to managing time better. These range from small clinics to big hospitals. Optimized time utilization allows caregivers to treat more patients and frees hospital testing rooms and beds for high volumes of patients. Without adequate caregivers and available rooms, some patients may die while waiting for their turns [2]. Figure 1, which shows these healthcare system principles for resource optimization.

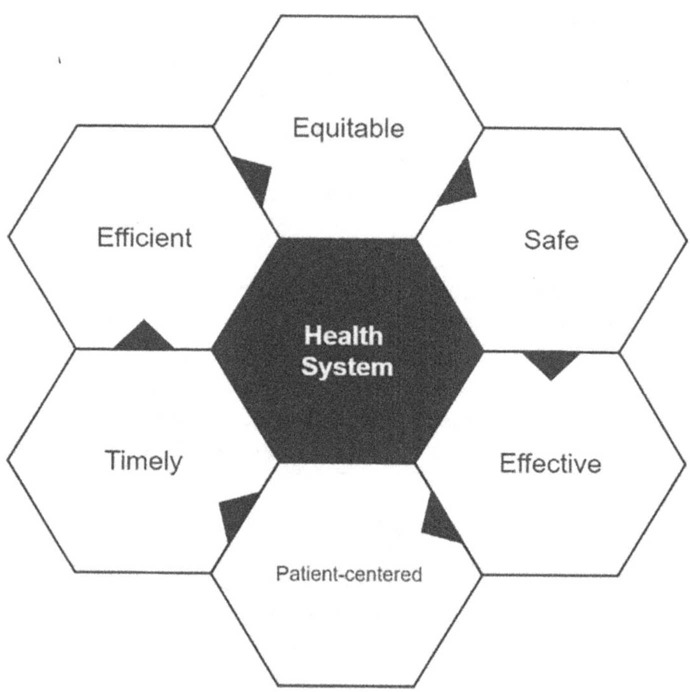

Fig. 1 Healthcare system principles

Figure 1 demonstrates that healthcare providers are obligated to prevent harm and deliver advantageous care to their patients. Services must be based on scientific evidence and provided to individuals who can gain benefits while preventing both underutilization and overutilization of resources. In addition, they must consider each patient's preferences, needs, and values when creating their care plan, acknowledging that capacities differ by gender, race, nationality, and socioeconomic status [3].

1.4 Principles of Effective Resource Management in Healthcare Systems

Today's healthcare systems encounter distinct challenges, highlighting the importance of managing resources effectively. Finding ways to make the most of limited resources in the face of growing demands can support healthcare professionals and enhance patient care. To bridge the gap between the ideal qualities of healthcare and current practices, the Institute of Medicine (IOM) panel suggested several actions aimed at enhancing efficiency, patient-centeredness, and safety for everyone involved in healthcare [2]. These actions are intended to improve the overall quality of healthcare delivery.

1. **Continuous Healing Relationships**

A better healthcare experience appears to depend on offering treatment whenever it is required in different forms. Offer treatment whenever needed and in various forms beyond the doctor's office visit, such as online consultations, phone calls, or other means, to make care more convenient for patients. The healthcare system is ready for patients 24/7, improving accessibility and resource utilization.

2. **Customizing Based on Patient Needs**

It is crucial that each patient receives customized care that fits their specific needs. Because every patient has a unique history, their treatment should be personalized to achieve better outcomes. Every patient is different; hence their treatment should represent that. This implies that healthcare should be customized to satisfy particular preferences as well as general requirements of every person. Healthcare may become more fit for the demands of both patients and physicians by emphasizing what people want and need.

3. **Patient as the Source of Control**

Comprehensive information is needed to empower patients to make treatment decisions for effective resource management. When patients get all the knowledge they need, they appear more suited to make choices about their treatment. Giving them this knowledge enables them to take charge and make decisions most fit for their circumstances.

4. **Shared Knowledge and Information Flow**

Maintaining open channels of contact between patients and their doctors would help all the participants to remain informed and make more wise choices together. The entire process of treating patients is quicker and more successful when patients can readily access their medical records and when doctors are free to share their expertise.

5. **Evidence-Based Decision-Making (EBDM)**

It is important for resource management to make decisions based on the best available evidence. This makes sure that patients get the best treatments and the same level of care no matter where they go or who they see.

6. **Prioritizing Patient Safety**

Healthcare providers should prioritize patient safety and integrate it into the system rather than treating it as an afterthought to reduce errors and protect patients. Minimizing costs and risks improves resource efficiency.

7. **Transparency in Information**

Patients must receive all necessary information to make informed choices regarding their treatments, health insurance, hospital procedures, and options. Transparency builds trust and eliminates unnecessary procedures, thereby conserving both financial resources and time in healthcare.

8. **Transparency in Healthcare**

Patients should possess all the knowledge required to make wise decisions about their treatment. Transparency in health insurance, hospitals, and treatment choices refers to ensuring that patients and their families may make the best selections possible by means of freely available information.

9. **Anticipation of Patient Needs**

Health care facilities should be ready to handle issues as they arise and try to ascertain what their patients might need before they really demand it. This proactive approach speeds up and facilitates more effective therapy. Reducing waste benefits everyone since it helps to lower costs and raise general quality of living by improving the treatment standards.

10. **Healthcare Provider Collaboration**

Encouragement of collaboration among physicians, nurses, and other healthcare workers would help the system to guarantee that patients get well-coordinated and complete treatment that covers all their requirements.

Figure 2 illustrates these concepts as a Mind Map of Key Strategies for Optimizing Healthcare, establishing a healthcare resource optimization framework abstracted from the IOM panel criteria.

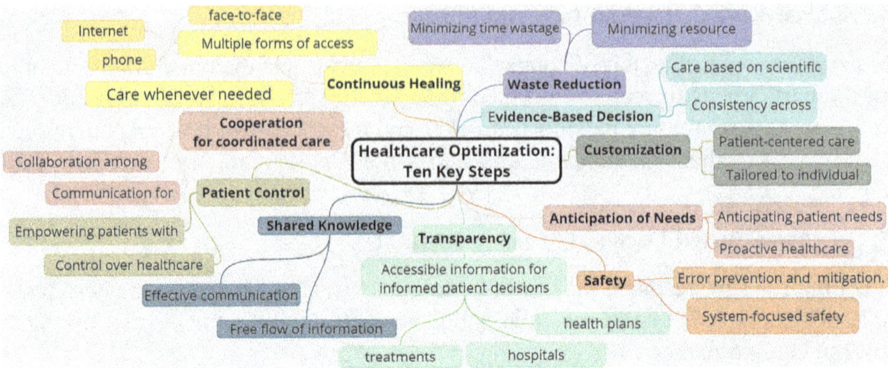

Fig. 2 Mind map of key strategies for optimizing healthcare

2 Generative Artificial Intelligence (GenAI)

From the moment we open our eyes to this world, the learning journey begins for gaining knowledge or skills through education or experience that comes from instinct or our capacity to create, either for survival, development of relationships, or the improvement of societal and personal conditions to help us taking proper decisions about current or future actions or reflect on past actions to enhance future performance.

If we are to claim that we have developed a machine capable of intelligence comparable to that of a human, generative modeling must be an integral part of that accomplishment. One of the clearest examples of a generative model in nature is the person engaging with this text. Pause for a moment to recognize the extraordinary generative model you are. You can visualize how sunlight filters through the trees in a sprawling forest at different times of day or fore-see different endings to a story you have written in your mind, or you can plan your week by envisioning various possible outcomes and adjusting your actions accordingly [4].The functions of the human brain have inspired experts to models that can have fundamentally similar performance to produce novel data that accurately reflect original data.

Generative artificial intelligence (GenAI) is a branch of machine learning that focuses on creating algorithms [5] that can mimic the features of training input data to make new, synthetic data that is different from the training data instead of gathered from actual events or observations. As opposed to other AI models, GenAI's goal is to generate rather than just make predictions or categorize.

To understand how generative AI works, consider it like an artist who studies the style and techniques of other artists. After spending time learning from various art pieces, the artist does not just copy them; instead, they create their own paintings that have similar styles, techniques, or themes but are entirely new and original. This novelty is what makes GenAI so intriguing. The reason Investigators have efforts to enhance computer intelligence to improve people's lives by developing or creating various algorithms and model topologies for their process of performance with tasks and data that can be classified from traditional methods like support vector machines (SVM) and decision trees (DT) to more advanced techniques like deep learning, which enables models to understand complex patterns in unstructured data through multiple processing layers, such as neural networks.Adopting the power of Generative AI is the most promising route to transform healthcare systems. It offers different benefits and a unique chance to improve medical treatments' accuracy, effectiveness, and speed. GANs can fundamentally change numerous fields, including resource allocation and medical treatment. Comprehending the methodologies underlying the most effective Generative AI models is vital for fully leveraging this potential. These include Variational Autoencoders (VAEs), Generative Adversarial Networks (GANs), Transformer-Based Generative Models, Flow-Based Models, and Diffusion Models, among others; each of these models reflects a distinct aspect of what segment of healthcare resources is best fit for every one of them, and explore practical approaches to using these models.

This chapter will go in-depth on several forms of Generative AI models, with particular attention on their applications to maximize resources in healthcare systems. Examining the ideas, uses, and difficulties related to every model helps us to offer complete knowledge that will help practitioners, scientists, and legislators to properly use these technologies.

2.1 Types of GenAI Models in Healthcare Resource Optimization

2.1.1 Variational Autoencoders (VAEs) Implementation

As Artificial Intelligence (AI) continues to advance, there is a clear trend toward incorporating AI into Computer-Aided Diagnosis (CAD) systems for both patients and healthcare providers. Many AI models depend on having access to high-quality training data to work well [6]. However, Acquiring a significant volume of medical data for CAD presents challenges due to the sensitive nature of the personal information contained within. As a result, there is a continual endeavor to investigate the utilization of generative models for the production of medical data.

VAEs integrate probabilistic reasoning and deep learning to acquire a condensed representation of data. These techniques are attractive because they are constructed using conventional function approximators (neural networks) and stochastic gradient descent for creating diverse and intricate data, such as handwritten medical records, facial symptoms of patients, numerical indicators of bodily conditions, physical models of medical scenarios, segmentation of diagnostic images, and forecasting future health outcomes based on static patient data [7]. These models illustrate their capability to produce medical images for improving research and diagnostics. They utilize a generative model within active learning to enhance the efficacy of classification models, prioritizing the proposed framework over the criteria for queries and enhancing the training dataset for labeling [8].

The complexity of the connections between the dimensions directly affects the difficulty of training generative models. For instance, producing visual representations of medical imaging data that demonstrate different anatomical structures in MRI scans is challenging. If one image segment depicts a portion of the lung, the adjacent section cannot simultaneously represent a part of the liver, as this would result in an anatomically incorrect image. It is crucial for the model to determine the structure before assigning values to individual pixels in the image. This type of decision is formally termed a latent variable (z) identification.

For instance, in a system that system monitors patient vitals and predicts critical pressure levels on a 0–9 scale, if a system part predicts a pressure level of 5, the output cannot include a 0, as this would be unrealistic or inaccurate. The model must first assess the patient's current condition before assigning prediction values. This decision-making process, known as latent variable identification, is critical for generating accurate predictions [7].

Unlike other methods, VAEs seek to create a correspondence between the input data and a probability distribution throughout the latent space. More precisely, the distribution is characterized by the mean and spread of a Gaussian distribution, which is commonly used for latent space sampling to help the produced output to be used as input for the decoder component, thereby enabling the model to generate new data [1]. VAEs are pretty helpful for tasks involving patient classification based on medical imaging data, risk assessment, and anomaly identification [9]. This efficiency is essential when healthcare resources are limited and when patient confidentiality must be protected by generating synthetic datasets instead of using accurate patient data [3].

Figure 3 depicts a VAE architecture, demonstrating how the encoder converts the initial input data into latent spaces (z). The transformation entails the computation of the Gaussian distribution's mean (μ) and standard deviation (σ). The latent variable z is generated by combining the parameters μ and σ with a random variable ε sampled from a Unit Gaussian Distribution. The lower-dimensional latent

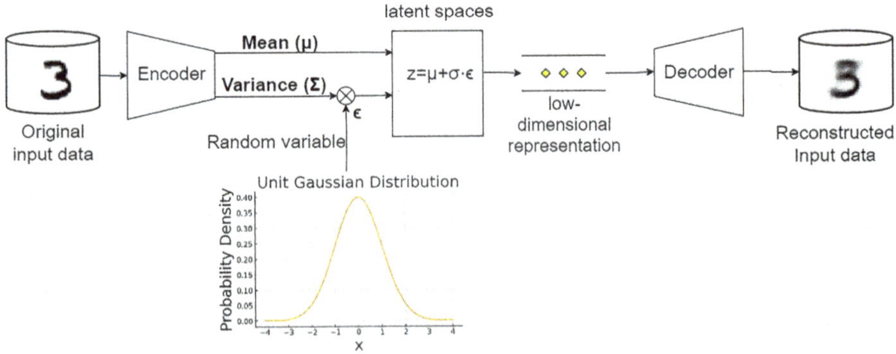

Fig. 3 Basic VAE architecture

representation is subsequently fed into the decoder, generative model, which reconstructs the data to its original form while maintaining crucial features for accurate reconstructions.

Mapping input data into a lower-dimensional space makes the vector preparable for mathematical operations(algorithms). For instance, a VAE objective is to capture an image of a sad person and then transform their mood to a state of happiness. First, the model finds a vector in latent space that specifies the direction of grin enhancement to compute the disparity between the mean positions of encoded images with and without smiling attributes in the latent space for calculating the grin vector. It can get a happier image after encoding the old image in latent space and changing it to a vector [3].

Applications of VAEs in Healthcare Resource Optimization

VAEs are an excellent technique for dealing with challenges for early diagnosis and risk assessment in clinical settings, which is one of the most important criteria In the medical domain [10]. Artificial patient data produced with VAEs can preserve patient secrecy while maintaining the statistical properties of real patient data. Then, especially in situations when the current actual data is limited or private, this artificially produced data can be utilized for training other machine learning models. Moreover, VAE is helpful in analyzing and generating complex datasets and helping identify abnormalities in healthcare systems, specifically about service receivers. Training a VAE on a dataset of healthy people will teach the model about approved data, so if there is a problem with the health system or a different parameter in patients' conditions, the system's functioning will recognize it.

Table 1 presents a comparison between traditional models and variational autoencoders (VAEs).

2.1.2 Generative Adversarial Networks (GANs) Implementation

Data collection presents a significant challenge for researchers and experts, particularly in the fields of medical data, due to privacy and confidentiality concerns that necessitate specific considerations. Sharing this information aids in validating experiments and enhancing comprehension of the facts [11]. Data de-identification is a viable method for sharing information while preserving privacy. However, this method primarily raises concerns about the potential to reverse the process and disclose the true identities of actual patients. Incentivizing patient populations to share data through rewards or benefits for their communities provides an additional data-sharing method [12]. This may be a feasible solution for small health ecosystems, but its scalability is uncertain. Each patient among the various stakeholders may have differing perceptions of issues, making consensus difficult to achieve [13].

Fundamentally, most machine learning projects assume that data samples are taken from a distinct data-generating distribution [14]. Generative models seek to learn this distribution utilizing several statistical learning techniques. Once the data-generating distribution is learned, we can create fresh data samples that differ from

Table 1 Comparative analysis of traditional models and VAEs

Aspect	Traditional models	VAEs
Data representation	Direct mapping from input to output, often rigid and predefined	Encodes input into a latent space, capturing key features in a compact, flexible form
Handling of complex data	Limited in handling high-dimensional and unstructured data, such as medical images or genomic data	Capable of efficiently managing high-dimensional, unstructured data by learning data distributions
Generative capabilities	Lacks the ability to generate new data; primarily used for prediction or classification tasks	Generates new data samples, simulating realistic patient data, useful for data augmentation and synthetic dataset creation
Anomaly detection	Typically relies on predefined thresholds and labels, limiting the ability to detect novel or rare anomalies	Learns the distribution of normal data, enabling the detection of anomalies through deviations in reconstruction error
Data privacy	Requires large amounts of real-world data, potentially exposing sensitive patient information	Can generate synthetic patient data, maintaining the statistical properties of real data while protecting patient privacy
Optimization in healthcare	Uses static models and predefined rules for resource allocation, limiting adaptability	Enables dynamic optimization through real-time learning of data patterns, improving resource allocation and patient outcomes

the input data, though not always exactly. Therefore, generative models can be considered safe tools for distributing new data while maintaining patient privacy [13].

GANs have garnered significant attention in both academia and the business world because they are resistant to overfitting and excel at modeling complex and high-dimensional data distributions across various data types [15], including images, audio, and others, and They have achieved exceptional performance in various image generation tasks, encompassing text-to-image synthesis, super-resolution [9], and image-to-image translation [3], which is particularly important in healthcare, where real data is often limited due to privacy reasons [16].

In Fig. 3, a GAN model comprises two neural networks. One of them is a discriminator for differentiating between authentic and generated data and one generator for producing synthetic data. The adversarial interaction between both networks enhances their performance, resulting in more realistic generated data (Fig. 4).

However, when dealing with big datasets or high-resolution outputs, GANs encounter difficulties like training instability. Resolutions are often critical for medical image generation, but they also increase the challenge and the likelihood of training failures. In addition, instability occurs because smaller batches are required due to memory constraints on GPUs.

Recent advancements in generative models have facilitated their effective integration into various other research disciplines. The objective of GAN models is to estimate data distributions (p-model) that closely align with the real distribution

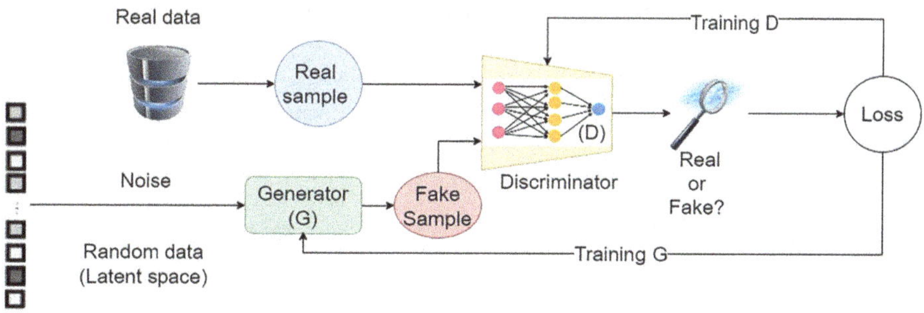

Fig. 4 Basic GANs architecture

(p-data). When estimating density, two primary issues must be taken into account. First, it is essential to select an appropriate objective function for the model. Second, it is required to ascertain the most effective p-model formulation that enhances the performance of generative models while facilitating efficient learning [17].

Challenges and Stability Issues in GANs

GANs sometimes suffer from training instability when working with high-resolution outputs or big datasets. Furthermore, instability can arise from the necessity for smaller batch sizes, usually determined by hardware constraints, especially GPU memory [18]. Moreover, mode collapse, characterized by the generator yielding a restricted variety of outputs, decreases the model's efficacy, represents another substantial challenge. In order to overcome these problems, new methods have been developed, like Wasserstein GANs (WGANs), which alter the learning process and produce outputs that are more stable and consistent.

Applications of GANs in Medical Imaging

When accurate patient data is unavailable or subject to privacy regulations because of the creation of synthetic datasets essential for training AI models, GANs play a crucial role in healthcare, particularly in improving medical imaging datasets [17, 19].

Generative AI can produce synthetic MRI or CT scans that replicate authentic images, thereby augmenting the reliability of diagnostic instruments trained on these datasets, or it can be used in fields such as oncology, where acquiring extensive datasets with varied pathological cases can be challenging [19].

Table 2 shows that generative AI, especially when GANs and VAEs are used, has greatly improved many healthcare applications. These models are very important for improving diagnoses, tailoring treatments to each person, and optimizing healthcare resources.

Table 2 Applications of GANs and VAEs in healthcare optimization

Healthcare area	GANs (generative adversarial networks)	VAEs (variational autoencoders)
Medical image creation	Generate synthetic images for training AI models (e.g., MRIs, CTs)	Create realistic images while preserving patient privacy
Anomaly detection	Identify anomalies by generating variations in data	Detect deviations from "normal" patient data patterns
Data augmentation	Expand datasets with diverse synthetic examples	Generate new data variations for improved AI training
Outcome prediction	Simulate various treatment outcomes for personalization	Predict health outcomes from patient data patterns
Privacy preservation	Generate synthetic data to protect patient privacy	Create anonymized data while retaining essential statistics
Drug discovery	Simulate drug interactions and molecular structures	Analyze drug data with simplified, compressed representations
Personalized medicine	Model treatment responses for tailored care	Profile patients for individualized treatment plans
Resource optimization	Simulate hospital flow to optimize staffing and bed management	Model resource allocation needs based on patient flow
Medical report generation	Generate automated, detailed medical reports	Summarize patient data for clear report generation

2.1.3 Low-Based Models Implementation

The flow-based Models category involves adaptation by altering the core or shared parameters to accommodate distributional disparities between domains. Highly accurate data observations from flow-based generative models and exact likelihood models help models to imply fast sampling and inference [20]. Although flow-based models offer improved computational efficiency, a crucial factor in healthcare environments where real-time data processing is vital, they usually show worse performance in density estimates in comparison to other approaches. Accurate likelihood estimation and smooth data reconstruction in both forward (data-to-noise) and backward (noise-to-data) processes depend on their ability to translate data into latent variable spaces via invertible transformations. For healthcare uses, including diagnosis imaging and real-time patient health monitoring, flow-based models mainly help when one can effectively manage massive datasets [7, 8] without sacrificing speed or accuracy.

Workflow and Architecture of Flow-Based Models

Flow-based models are built on a series of invertible transformations that streamline complex data distributions into latent spaces, allowing them to compress and handle complex medical datasets more efficiently. Techniques like real-valued non-volume preserving (RealNVP) transformations are frequently employed in this procedure because of their efficient data processing ability and ability to ensure the model's scalability [8]. The incorporation of coupling layers in its architecture ensures that transformations are invertible, permitting a segment of the data to remain unaltered while the remainder is transformed.

Figure 5 illustrates the general workflow of a flow-based model, from the initial input data (X) through its transformation into a simplified latent space, followed by the inverse transformations and the reconstruction of the original data (X′).

Applications of DM in Precision Medicine and Resource Optimization
Flow-based models are highly suitable for precision medicine, because they excel in accurately modeling data, which is crucial for understanding and customizing therapy for specific patients and enhances patient care standards and optimizes resource use by reducing the strain on medical equipment and healthcare staff. Additionally, this method improves operational scalability while ensuring accuracy and facilitates the management of more complex datasets. The effective architecture of these models is essential for resource optimization, particularly in hospitals managing diverse patient data in real-time [7]. Physicians can improve treatment personalization by employing new data and minimizing unnecessary interventions.

2.1.4 Diffusion Models Implementation

Diffusion Models (DMs) are a class of generative models that systematically introduce and eliminate noise to understand the fundamental distribution of training data for data generation. They are designed using deep neural networks and stochastic processes to estimate the score of a data distribution. Simulating the forward Stochastic Differential Equation (SDE) adds noise to data. In the opposite process, neural networks eliminate noise to provide high-quality samples that match the original data to comprehend the fundamental distribution of the training data [15].

In Fig. 6, the general pipeline of a DM comprises three primary phases: the forward process, in which noise is incrementally added to the training data to characterize its distribution; the reverse process, wherein noise is eliminated to produce new data to enable the model to acquire knowledge of the underlying data structure incrementally; and the sampling process, where a random noise sample serves as the input, and the network systematically reverses the noise through a sequence of time-indexed steps. In this process, stochastic differential equations (SDEs) balance theoretical frameworks and practical applications.

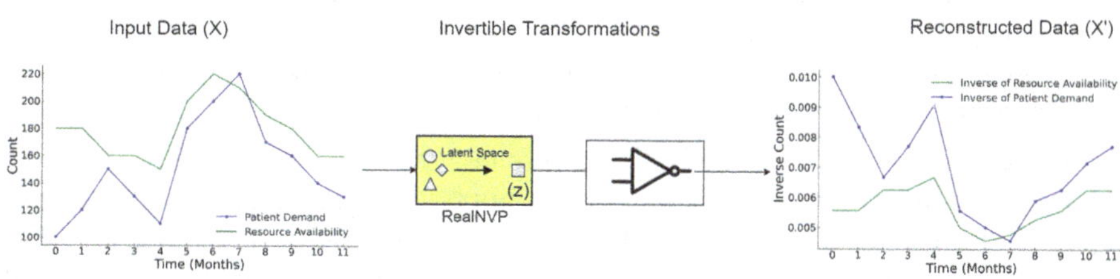

Fig. 5 Flow-based model architecture

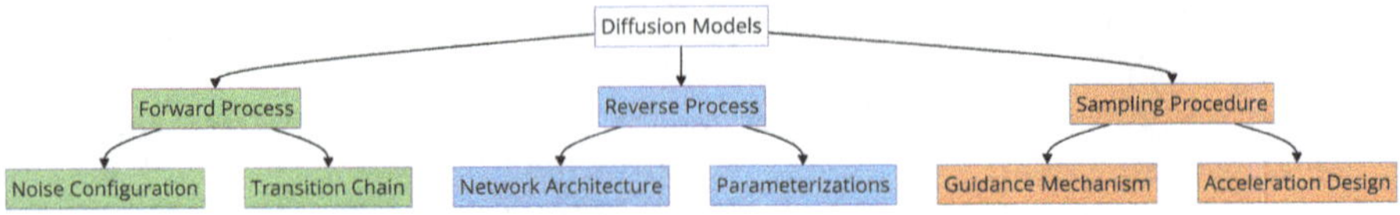

Fig. 6 Key components of diffusion models

Applications of DMs in Precision Medicine and Healthcare Resource Optimization

DMs are flexible and suitable for various medical data types, including images, genomic sequences, and patient monitoring data, enabling a wide range of healthcare applications. They also protect patient privacy by generating synthetic patient data for machine learning model training and allow healthcare systems to simulate realistic medical conditions using noisy data to improve medical imaging quality with high-fidelity data [16].

Despite the growing significance of DMs, the literature persists in not thoroughly examining their design principles. Much of the research primarily concentrates on particular components, such as the forward and reverse processes, or specifically targets individual applications [16].

In precision medicine, decision-makers excel at managing a variety of data types, enabling the analysis of medical history, genomic data, and real-time monitoring to develop personalized treatment strategies that optimize healthcare resource allocation to ensure effective resource use. DMs improve medical imaging quality and generate high-resolution synthetic images, which improves diagnostic accuracy. This improves healthcare decisions, reduces unnecessary procedures, and optimizes resource use [16].

2.1.5 Transformer-Based Generative Models Implementation

Present investigations and various clinical applications extensively utilize Electronic Health Records (EHRs), which represent both categorized structured data and unstructured clinical text. Organizing clinical text effectively to extract patient information presents a significant challenge in the utilization of Electronic Health Records (EHRs) [21]. Clinical narratives serve as the primary method for documenting essential patient information, including medical history, adverse medication events, and social, behavioral, and environmental factors influencing an individual's health. Identifying significant clinical concepts from clinical report text has been a primary focus of detailed exploration in Natural Language Processing (NLP) techniques and resources [22]. Various natural language processing architectures have been developed and examined to improve the accuracy of clinical concept extraction, including rule-based, machine learning, and hybrid models [23]. The rise of deep learning models has led to a notable shift in the study of clinical concept extraction.

Although many studies have examined transformer-based models for clinical applications on a case-by-case basis, there remains a deficiency in comprehensive exploration and comparison of their performance in the biomedical field. Moreover, there is a lack of packages featuring pre-trained clinical transformers that could assist individuals in utilizing these advanced NLP models for a range of downstream clinical NLP tasks. Their ability to manage intricate data sequences, including patient records and medical histories, enables them to produce medical reports and forecast patient outcomes with impressive precision [24]. The attention mechanisms in these models allow for a concentration on the most significant elements of the data, thereby improving their effectiveness in tasks like report generation and clinical decision support [25].

The figure below illustrates how transformers operate on healthcare data, enabling the generation of medical reports and the execution of predictive analysis (Fig. 7).

Applications of Transformer-Based Models in Resource Optimization
Transformer-based generative models adeptly analyze sequential data, such as patient health records, to emphasize critical data points, ensuring that medical reports are comprehensive and pertinent to the context [24, 25].

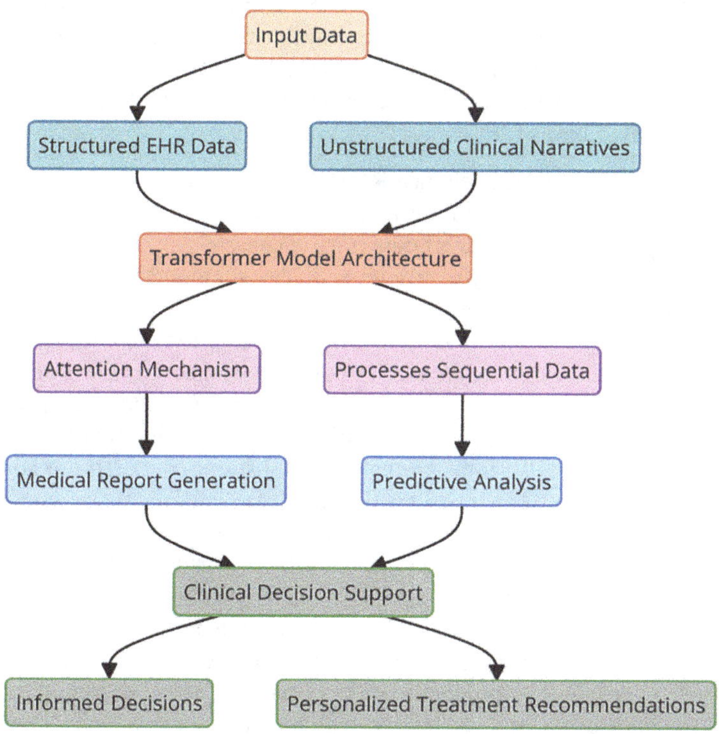

Fig. 7 Transformer models in healthcare data processing

Healthcare professionals can prioritize patient care over report writing, optimizing the utilization of human resources. On the other hand, Transformers identify patterns and correlations in patient records that assist physicians in determining treatment strategies and resource allocation. This ability to predict helps decide what resources are needed, like staff and supplies, which speeds up processes. Transformers can also help people make decisions by giving them advice based on facts, lowering the chance of mistakes, and ensuring that resources are used in the best way possible [25].

2.1.6 Energy-Based Models (EBMs)

The main objective of statistical modeling and machine learning is to illustrate the connections among variables. Capturing these dependencies allows a model to answer questions regarding the values of unknown variables and unseen data based on the values of known variables [26].

Energy-based models (EBMs) can be considered a class of generative models that learn input data and represent these dependencies by assigning a scalar energy value, which serves as a metric for compatibility with each variable configuration.

Compared to traditional models, EBMs do not necessitate normalization across the entire space. They depend on relative energy differences rather than absolute probabilities, rendering them especially appropriate for high-dimensional data prevalent in healthcare applications. This approach allows EBMs to clarify the fundamental structure of the data without the computational burden of normalizing across all possible configurations [26].

Applications of EBMs in Healthcare Resource Optimization

EBMs are especially effective in modeling complex systems in healthcare where several interdependent factors affect outcomes. Their capacity to capture dependencies without explicit probability distributions makes them ideally suited for various uses in healthcare resource optimization.

EBM models assist hospitals in detecting demand anomalies by analyzing the energy landscape based on patient admissions, bed occupancy, and staffing levels. This analysis ensures that facilities are adequately staffed and equipped to meet patient needs, resulting in a practical solution for optimizing healthcare resource allocation [27]. Conversely, conventional probabilistic models require administrators to assess and normalize every conceivable resource allocation configuration among departments, including the Emergency Room (ER), Intensive Care Unit (ICU), and General Ward, to estimate probabilities for each scenario. This method rapidly becomes computationally unmanageable as the number of potential configurations increases, rendering it ineffective for real-time decision-making [26].

In addition, EBMs help hospital managers reduce energy consumption across several departments. Due to a higher number of patients, the Emergency Room usually exhibits more urgency and activity, calling for more resources. By contrast, departments like the General Ward, which have less activity, require fewer resources.

Providing resources to reduce energy consumption in the areas with the most significant demand improves the distribution of resources, even without normalization [28]. By focusing on specific areas, we can improve efficiency and ensure that the most important departments to patients get the resources they need to stay well.

2.1.7 Autoregressive Models

Autoregressive models are a significant class of generative models that decompose a dataset's joint probability distribution into a sequence of conditional probabilities. Predicting future values based on preceding ones is particularly effective for sequential data and time-series analysis, which are essential in healthcare applications [29].

Time-series models based on deep learning have become popular because they can train global models end-to-end, integrate external covariates effortlessly, and automatically extract relevant features [30]. Often, individual time series within a dataset are statistically dependent on each other to produce accurate predictions. This inductive bias should ideally be incorporated into deep learning models through the use of multivariate probabilistic methods [31].

Recent advancements in generation tasks, encompassing audio, text, image, and video, have been achieved by applying convolutional autoregressive models, notably WaveNet and PixelCNN. Rapid, parallel training methodologies, which are essential to their success, significantly enhance the effectiveness of these models [29]. However, the generation process can be prolonged for practical use due to unnecessary repetitions of irrelevant calculations [29]. In this model, the utilization of cached previously computed hidden states has decreased computational complexity, enhancing autoregressive models' efficiency in clinical contexts that require prompt predictions.

Applications of Autoregressive Models in Healthcare Resource Optimization
Autoregressive models utilize historical data to predict patient vital signs or medical conditions, enhancing real-time healthcare decision-making.

During pandemics, multivariate autoregressive models clarify the relationships between resources, including personnel, equipment, and patient admissions, resulting in more accurate predictions and enhanced resource management [32]. Moreover, these models tackle data collection challenges by quantifying the necessary data for precise resource need forecasting. At the same time, continuous advancements in statistical and machine-learning techniques seek to enhance these predictions [33].

Methods often resort to using tractable distribution classes or low-rank approximations to model the full predictive distribution, regardless of the actual data distribution. However, probabilistic methods with tractable likelihoods are necessary to accurately and generally model the data distribution. Several deep learning approaches, such as autoregressive models [34] and generative models based on normalizing flows [35], have been proposed to learn flexible models of high-dimensional multivariate time series.

Even when the full likelihood is not tractable, a tractable lower bound to the probability can often be optimized. However, these methods require specific structures in the functional approximators, such as constraints on the determinant of the Jacobian for normalizing flows [36]. In contrast, Energy-Based Models (EBMs), as previously discussed, have a less restrictive functional form. They approximate the unnormalized log probability, In contrast, Energy-Based Models (EBMs), as previously discussed, have a less restrictive functional form. They approximate the unnormalized log probability, thereby transforming density estimation into a nonlinear regression problem. EBMs exhibit robust capabilities in learning high-dimensional data distributions; however, their training can be complex [26, 37].

Autoregressive models possess inherent limitations. A notable limitation is that standard autoregressive models execute only polynomial-time computations to forecast the probability of the subsequent symbol. While this computational efficiency is advantageous for training and sampling, it means that these models struggle to represent distributions where the next-symbol probability is hard to compute [38].

Consequently, autoregressive models cannot adequately capture certain complex distributions, limiting their expressiveness. They may fail to model distributions well enough to solve associated decision problems that practitioners might encounter in healthcare analytics. These limitations persist regardless of the amount of computation and data used during training unless the model parameters grow super-polynomially with sequence length, which is impractical [38].

Autoregressive models are optimally designed for probability distributions that allow for the efficient computation of prefix probabilities. While this efficiency is advantageous, it inherently restricts the model's capacity to represent more intricate distributions unless we permit computational time or model parameters to increase exponentially with input length [38]. This limitation poses a considerable issue in healthcare applications that involve lengthy sequences or necessitate modeling complex dependencies.

3 Conclusion

Including cutting-edge Generative AI models into medical systems has great potential to maximize resources, raise patient outcomes, and increase operational effectiveness. Models like Variational Autoencoders (VAEs), Generative Adversarial Networks (GANs), Flow-Based Models, and Diffusion Models can solve certain problems in healthcare because they have their own special skills. By generating new data, these models help to solve the problem of not having enough real data and protect patient privacy at the same time. This lets us make better diagnostic tools and personalized treatment plans. VAEs help make the different datasets that are needed to train machine learning models well, and GANs make high-quality medical images that help doctors make more accurate diagnoses. Flow-Based Models are great at processing data in real time, which is important in dynamic healthcare settings. Conversely, Diffusion Models employ sophisticated noise management techniques to ensure the generation of high-quality data, thereby reducing waste and enhancing the quality of care.

To solve interpretability, computational, and data management issues for the application of Generative AI in healthcare, technologists, doctors, and legislators must work together. One needs cooperation. Multidisciplinary to include Generative AI models into healthcare systems since of their complexity and data sensitivity. Computational challenges have to be solved if we are to guarantee these models operate in real-time healthcare. Through cross-field collaboration and advanced Generative AI models, healthcare companies can enhance predictive, tailored, and efficient delivery of treatment. This change can maximize operational processes and resource allocation, so delivering technological developments to society and individuals. Strategic integration produces an adaptive, flexible healthcare system.

References

1. Brandeau MLSF, Pierskalla WP. Operations research and health care: a handbook of methods and applications. Kluwer Academic Publishers; 2004.
2. Ferlay JA, et al. Preventing cancer through tobacco and infection control: lung cancer, cervical cancer, and stomach cancer. Eur J Cancer Prev. 2008;17(4) [Online]. Available: https://journals.lww.com/eurjcancerprev/abstract/2008/04000/preventing_cancer_through_tobacco_and_infection.12.aspx
3. Foster D. Generative deep learning: teaching machines to paint, write, compose, and play. 1st ed. O'Reilly Media; 2019.
4. Doersch C. Tutorial on variational autoencoders. Carnegie Mellon University/UC Berkeley; 2016. (with note for 2021 revision). [Online]. Available: https://arxiv.org/abs/1606.05908
5. Ángel Canal-Alonso NE, Jiménez P, Corchado JM. Revolutionizing pharmaceuticals: generative artificial intelligence as a bibliographic assistant. Carbajosa de la Sagrada: Department of Bioinformatics and Computational Biology, AIR Institute; 2021. [Online]. Available: http://hdl.handle.net/10366/153110
6. In-Gyu Lee J-YO, Hee-Jung Y, Kim J-H, Eom K-D, Je J-H. Generative active learning with variational autoencoder for radiology data generation in veterinary medicine. Singapore; 2024.
7. Ghayoumi M. Generative adversarial networks in practice. CRC Press; 2024. https://doi.org/10.1201/9781003281344.
8. Zhu CVX, Fowlkes CC, Ramanan D. Do we need more training data? arXiv Preprint, arXiv:1503.01508v1. 2015:1–22. https://doi.org/10.1007/s11263-015-0812-2.
9. Jia-Jie Zhu JB. Generative adversarial active learning. arXiv Preprint. 2017; https://arxiv.org/abs/1702.07956v5
10. Cao DSJ. Generative adversarial networks (GANs): challenges, solutions, and future directions. ACM Comput Surv. 2021;54(3):63. https://doi.org/10.1145/3446374.
11. Howard Bauchner MRMG, Fontanarosa B. Data sharing: an ethical and scientific imperative. JAMA J Am Med Assoc. 2016;315(12):1238–40. https://doi.org/10.1001/jama.2016.2420.
12. Matthew PSJ, McCoy S, Emanuel EJ. Sharing patient data without exploiting patients. JAMA J Am Med Assoc. 2020;323(6):505–6. https://doi.org/10.1001/jama.2019.22354.
13. Ayyoubzadeh SMASM, Esmaeili M. Clinical data sharing using generative adversarial networks. Connected Health. 2022;1:98–100. https://doi.org/10.20517/ch.2022.15.
14. Ian Goodfellow YB, Courville A. Deep learning. MIT Press; 2016.

15. Preeti Sharma MK, Sharma HK, Biju SM. Generative adversarial networks (GANs): introduction, taxonomy, variants, limitations, and applications. Multimed Tools Appl. 2024; https://doi.org/10.1007/s11042-024-18767-y.
16. Laurent Dinh DK, Bengio Y. Non-linear independent components estimation. In: Presented at the 4th international conference on learning representations (ICLR '15) workshop; 2015.
17. Liu MYTO. Coupled generative adversarial networks. In: Presented at the Advances in Neural Information Processing Systems, 2016. [Online]. Available: https://arxiv.org/abs/1606.07536.
18. Mahmoud Ibrahim YAK, Amirrajab S, Sun C, Breeuwer M, Pluim J, Elen B, Dumontier M, Ertaylan G. Generative AI for synthetic data across multiple medical modalities: a systematic review of recent developments and challenges. arXiv Preprint. 2024; https://doi.org/10.48550/arXiv.2407.00116.
19. Chang ZK, Shum G, Hubert PH. On the design fundamentals of diffusion models: a survey. ArXiv Preprint. 2023; [Online]. Available: https://arxiv.org/abs/2306.04542v3
20. Homayoun Safarpour MM, Farhadi A, Molnár G, Nagy E. Generative adversarial networks for heterogeneous unsupervised domain adaptation detection. In: Presented at the IEEE 28th international conference on intelligent engineering systems (INES 2024). Gammarth; 2024.
21. Yanshan Wang LW, Rastegar-Mojarad M, Moon S, Shen F, Afzal N, Liu S, Zeng Y, Mehrabi S, Sohn S, Liu H. Clinical information extraction applications: a literature review. J Biomed Inform. 2018;77:34–49.
22. Sunyang Fu DC, He H, Liu S, Moon S, Peterson KJ, Shen F, Wang L, Wang Y, Wen A, Zhao Y, Sohn S, Liu H. Development of clinical concept extraction applications: a methodology review. arXiv Preprint. 2020; https://doi.org/10.48550/arXiv.1910.11377.
23. James Masanz SVP, Xu H, Wu ST, Chute CG, Liu H. Open source clinical NLP – more than any single system. 2014.
24. Ian Goodfellow JP-A, Mirza M, Bing X, Warde-Farley D, Ozair S, Courville A, Bengio Y. Generative adversarial networks. Commun ACM. 2020;63(11):139–44. https://doi.org/10.1145/3422622.
25. Xi Yang JB, Hogan WR, Yonghui W. Clinical concept extraction using transformers. J Am Med Inform Assoc. 2020;27(12):1935–42. https://doi.org/10.1093/jamia/ocaa189.
26. Yann LeCun SC, Hadsell R, Ranzato M'A, Huang FJ. In: Bakir THG, Schölkopf B, Smola A, Taskar B, editors. A tutorial on energy-based learning. MIT Press; 2006. p. 191–246.
27. Shuangfei Zhai YC, Lu W, Zhang Z(M). Deep structured energy based models for anomaly detection. In: Presented at the proceedings of the 33rd international conference on machine learning (ICML). New York; 2016.
28. Oumaima Manchadi F-EB-B, Jioudi B. Predictive maintenance in healthcare systems: a survey. IEEE Access. 2022; https://doi.org/10.1109/ACCESS.2023.3287490.
29. Prajit Ramachandran BZ, Le QV. Searching for activation functions. arXiv Preprint. 2017; https://arxiv.org/abs/1710.05941
30. Konstantinos Benidis SSR, Flunkert V, Wang Y, Maddix DC, Türkmen AC, Gasthaus J, Bohlke-Schneider M, Salinas D, Stella L, Callot L, Januschowski T. Neural forecasting: introduction and literature overview. arXiv Preprint. 2020; https://arxiv.org/abs/2004.10240
31. Tsay RS. Multivariate time series analysis: with R and financial applications. Hoboken: Wiley; 2014.
32. Liang Chen YZ, Tang X, Dai Q. High-dimensional vector autoregressive models for forecasting healthcare time series. Appl Soft Comput. 2020;97:Art no 106770. https://doi.org/10.1016/j.asoc.2020.106770.
33. Galit Shmueli OK. Predictive analytics in information systems research. MIS Q. 2011;35(3):553–72. https://hdl.handle.net/1765/87835
34. Aaron van den Oord NK, Espeholt L, Kavukcuoglu K, Vinyals O, Graves A. Conditional image generation with PixelCNN decoders. In: Presented at the Advances in Neural Information Processing Systems (NeurIPS 2016); 2016. [Online]. Available: https://papers.nips.cc/paper/6527-conditional-image-generation-with-pixelcnn-decoders.

35. George Papamakarios EN, Rezende DJ, Mohamed S, Lakshminarayanan B. Normalizing flows for probabilistic modeling and inference. J Mach Learn Res. 2021;22:1–64. [Online]. Available: https://jmlr.org/papers/volume22/19-1028/19-1028.pdf
36. Laurent Dinh JS-D, Bengio S. Density estimation using real NVP. In: Presented at the international conference on learning representations (ICLR); 2017.
37. Hinton GE. Training products of experts by minimizing contrastive divergence. Neural Comput. 2002;14(8):1771–800. https://doi.org/10.1162/089976602760128018.
38. Chu-Cheng Lin AJ, Li X, Gormley MR, Eisner J. Limitations of autoregressive models and their alternatives. In: Proceedings of the 2021 conference of the North American Chapter of the Association for Computational Linguistics: Human Language Technologies (NAACL-HLT); 2021. p. 5147–73. https://doi.org/10.18653/v1/2021.naacl-main.405.

Ethics and Regulations in Generative AI

Armin ZadZiabari and Azadeh Tabatabaei

1 Introduction

With the rise of AI, the healthcare industry is undergoing a sea change. AI holds transformative potential in healthcare, such as diagnostics, personalized medicine, drug discovery, patient data management, and clinical decision-making [1]. This innovative technology employs natural language processing (NLP) and computer vision (CV) techniques to emulate human intelligence. As AI in healthcare advances, it presents a range of ethical and regulatory challenges that demand careful consideration. In data-driven healthcare, the protection of patient privacy is essential, as it has the potential to affect data sharing and psychological well-being. The transparency and reliability of AI systems are crucial, especially in high-stakes decision-making contexts. One essential component that has recently emerged is explainable AI (XAI), which ensures that predictions made by AI can be understood clearly.

Machine learning (ML), a subset of AI, enables algorithms to learn patterns from data without explicit programming. Deep learning (DL) is a subset of ML that employs multilayered artificial neural networks, allowing DL algorithms to represent and comprehend intricate data patterns effectively. These days, Generative artificial intelligence (GenAI) is rapidly transforming various domains, including healthcare. GenAI refers to a category of algorithms that can generate new data samples from learned distributions of input data. OpenAI ChatGPT, Google Gemini, and other competitors are also advanced large language models (LLMs) trained on

Both authors contributed equally.

A. ZadZiabari (✉) · A. Tabatabaei
Department of Computer Engineering, University of Science and Culture, Tehran, Iran
e-mail: arminzedu@gmail.com; a.tabatabaei@usc.ac.ir

A. Zamanifar, M. Faezipour (eds.), *Application of Generative AI in Healthcare Systems*, https://doi.org/10.1007/978-3-031-82963-5_8

extensive data to produce human-like responses to user inquiries. This potential in medicine, research, and education is significant (see Fig. 1).

The complexity of AI-generated decisions, particularly in life-critical areas like diagnostics and treatment recommendations, underscores the urgent need for accountability, transparency, and fairness. The opacity of many AI models, often referred to as black-box systems, raises concerns about the explainability of AI-driven medical decisions [2]. When clinical outcomes are influenced by models whose inner workings are not easily interpretable, the question of accountability becomes crucial, especially in cases of misdiagnosis or incorrect treatment recommendations. Furthermore, AI systems are often trained on large datasets, which introduces concerns regarding data privacy and patient confidentiality. Studies have shown that AI systems can unintentionally perpetuate biases present in the training data, leading to unequal treatment of minority populations [3]. These biases can manifest in various healthcare contexts, such as predicting disease risk or allocating resources, and they underline the critical need for fairness and equity in AI design and implementation. High-profile regulations, such as the Health Insurance Portability and Accountability Act (HIPAA) in the United States and the General Data Protection Regulation (GDPR) in Europe, impose strict controls over how personal health information is used and shared. However, as AI technologies evolve, these frameworks may prove insufficient to address the full spectrum of ethical and legal challenges.

Integrating GenAI into healthcare is also challenging due to the role of human emotions. Autonomous systems may not offer the same colleague consultations as

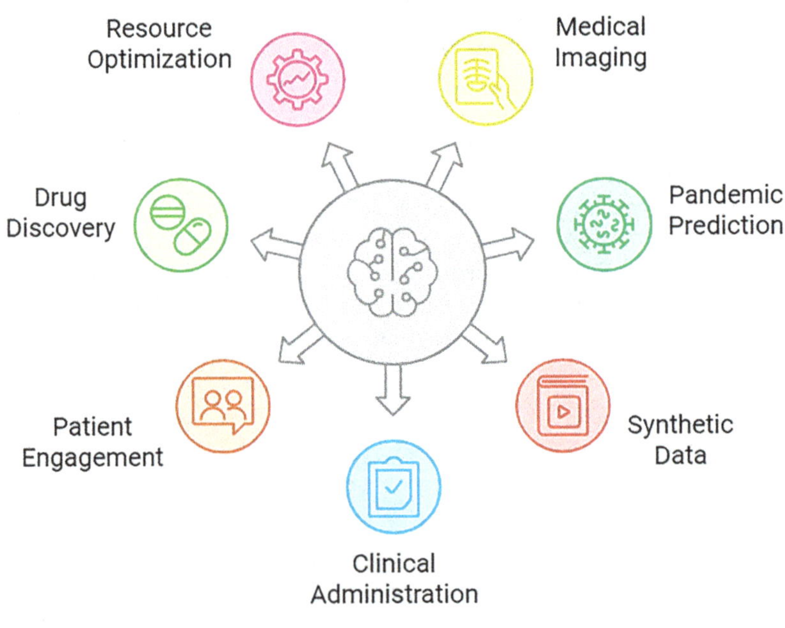

Fig. 1 Applications of Generative AI in Healthcare

medical professionals do. Compassion and empathy, which are essential for healing, may be lost with AI physicians and nurses, as they lack these human traits. This can be considered as a key limitation of AI in medical science.

2 Ethical Implications of Generative AI in Healthcare

2.1 Autonomy and Informed Consent

Patient autonomy is a cornerstone of medical ethics, ensuring that individuals make informed decisions about their health based on a clear understanding of their options. Generative AI (GenAI) systems, however, present unique challenges in this notion, especially with informed consent.

GenAI in healthcare presents significant challenges in ensuring individual autonomy and informed consent. These systems can influence medical decisions, potentially complicating the process of obtaining informed consent from patients. People may have trouble understanding the decision-making process due to the complicated nature of AI algorithms, which raises ethical questions about transparency and autonomy [4]. For informed consent to remain ethically sound in the context of GenAI, healthcare providers must ensure that both the risks and benefits of AI-based recommendations are communicated clearly and that patients retain control over their treatment choices.

2.2 Responsibility and Accountability

The growing reliance on GenAI raises critical questions about accountability. Who is responsible if an AI system provides a wrong diagnosis or treatment recommendation? The fact that these systems often operate semi-autonomously complicates the responsibility when mistakes occur [5]. Developers, healthcare providers, or the institutions that implement these technologies may be accountable. Establishing clear guidelines and frameworks is essential to ensure ethical AI implementation in healthcare [6]. The existing model often imposes the responsibility on clinicians, potentially reducing their role to merely validating AI decisions, which may result in ethical and legal challenges [7].

2.3 *Beneficence and Non-maleficence*

Healthcare AI systems in healthcare must adhere to the ethical principles of beneficence and non-maleficence, ensuring that they inflict no damage. Nonetheless, biases in AI algorithms may result in unintended harm, exacerbating health disparities and violating these principles [8]. AI systems should be continuously monitored in real-world settings to confirm that they maintain accuracy and do not introduce unintended biases over time [9]. Models trained on incomplete, biased, or unrepresentative data can also produce recommendations that perpetuate inequalities in care [3].

2.4 *Case-Based Ethical Insights*

AI systems have been successfully implemented in areas like radiology, where AI-assisted diagnostic tools have enhanced the accuracy of image-based diagnoses, reducing human error and improving patient outcomes [10]. The SENSOMATT project highlights ethical challenges in AI healthcare applications, particularly the importance of understanding data owner rights and establishing ethical norms for AI use in medical applications, especially in nursing [11]. GenAI has been utilized to optimize clinical documentation, reducing the burden on healthcare professionals. A case study demonstrated the use of AI to generate clinical notes, improving documentation quality and patient-centered care. Ethical considerations included maintaining patient confidentiality and addressing model biases [12]. Figure 2 illustrates the ethical implications of GenAI aspects in healthcare.

3 Privacy and Data Security in Generative AI for Healthcare

3.1 *Sensitive Nature of Medical Data*

Medical data is among the most sensitive forms of personal data, often containing detailed records of an individual's health status, genetic information, and treatment history. The sensitive nature of this data presents a significant challenge for healthcare providers and AI developers, as any misuse of medical information can result in severe consequences for patients. Generative adversarial networks (GANs) and large language models (LLMs) are increasingly used in healthcare for diagnostics, treatment planning, and research. These systems require extensive health data, raising significant privacy concerns. Protecting sensitive patient information is crucial, as breaches can lead to severe consequences, including identity theft and loss of trust in healthcare systems [13].

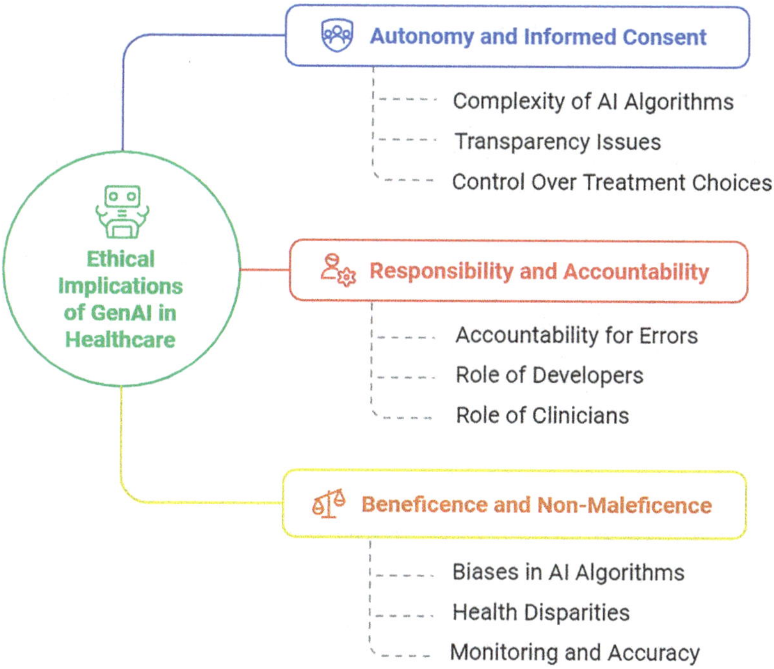

Fig. 2 Ethical implications of GenAI aspects in healthcare

3.2 Data Anonymization and De-identification

De-identification techniques have been adopted in AI healthcare applications to remove personally identifiable information (PII) from electronic health record (EHR) data, ensuring that individuals cannot be directly linked to their data. Anonymization, in particular, seeks to irreversibly modify data so that it cannot be traced back to any individual, while de-identification focuses on removing or masking key identifiers such as names, addresses, and social security numbers [14]. While these approaches are essential for protecting personal privacy, they are not without limitations. A key concern is the potential for re-identification, where anonymized data can be cross-referenced with other datasets to re-establish individual identities. Studies have shown that even when datasets are anonymized, the use of advanced machine learning techniques can sometimes allow for the re-identification of individuals based on seemingly innocuous data points, particularly in small or highly specific populations [15]. In some cases, the process of anonymization can strip away valuable information that is necessary for training effective AI models, reducing the overall performance and accuracy of these systems. Balancing the need for privacy with the need for high-quality, usable data remains an ongoing challenge in AI development.

3.3 Emerging Challenges in Data Security

Generative models, particularly those used in healthcare, are often targeted by attackers aiming to steal sensitive information or manipulate AI systems to produce erroneous outputs. Additionally, adversarial attacks pose a growing threat to the integrity of AI in healthcare. These attacks involve subtly altering an AI system's input data in ways that are imperceptible to humans but cause the AI to make incorrect predictions or decisions. In a healthcare context, this could lead to disastrous outcomes, such as the misclassification of medical images or faulty treatment recommendations [16]. Given these emerging challenges, healthcare organizations must adopt comprehensive security strategies that include encryption, robust access controls, and continuous monitoring of generative models. Enhancing transparency and conducting clinical validations are also essential to mitigate these risks [17].

4 Algorithmic Bias and Fairness of Generative AI in Healthcare

4.1 Understanding Bias in Generative Models

Bias in generative AI (GenAI) emerges from multiple stages in the AI lifecycle, including the acquisition of training data, the design of algorithms, and their implementation in practical healthcare environments. Training data is a foundational source of bias. Since AI models learn patterns from historical data, any pre-existing biases in the data, such as underrepresentation of certain groups or skewed healthcare outcomes based on race, gender, or socioeconomic status, are likely to be inherited by the AI system [18].

Beyond data, model design can also perpetuate bias. AI models are engineered to optimize particular outcomes, and the design decisions can unintentionally favor certain populations over others. Moreover, bias can emerge during deployment when AI systems are applied in contexts they were not trained for or when system feedback loops exacerbate initial disparities [19]. The compounding effect indicates that biases in GenAI are frequently nuanced, developing progressively as the AI engages with diverse populations, hence complicating detection and remediation efforts.

4.2 *Mitigating Bias in Gen AI*

A fundamental strategy for reducing bias in GenAI is data diversification. Ensuring that training datasets accurately represent various populations mitigates the risk of biased results. This involves collecting data from various demographic groups to ensure inclusivity and fairness in AI models [20].

Continuous auditing and monitoring of AI systems are essential to identify and mitigate biases over time. This involves regularly evaluating models to detect any emerging biases and implementing corrective measures. Transparency in AI processes and outcomes is vital to maintaining accountability and trust [21].

4.3 *Insights from Case Studies Analysis*

Several case studies highlight the ethical challenges posed by algorithmic bias in GenAI within healthcare. For instance, modifying latent space directions in text-to-image models can help create diverse and inclusive outputs without altering the original embeddings. This approach facilitates adaptable and precise bias reduction [22]. Another case was a generative model for medical imaging diagnostics, trained mostly on data from White patients, which showed performance gaps when diagnosing skin diseases in minority populations. Limited exposure to darker skin tones reduced its accuracy in detecting melanoma in Black and Hispanic patients [23].

These case studies highlight the ethical concerns of implementing biassed GenAI in healthcare and the requirement of constant awareness, testing, and updating of AI models to ensure that they provide fair health outcomes for all populations.

5 Explainability and Transparency in Generative Models

5.1 *The Role of Explainability in AI-Driven Care*

Explainability in generative AI (GenAI) models is crucial in healthcare due to the high stakes involved in medical decision-making. These models must be transparent to healthcare providers and patients to build trust and ensure informed decisions. The complexity of GenAI, such as GANs and large language models, often results in black box systems, which can hinder clinical adoption and patient confidence [24]. The lack of explainability complicates legal and ethical responsibilities. Transparent AI systems enable the tracing of decision-making processes, which is essential for addressing biases or errors. This accountability is crucial for ethical AI deployment in healthcare, ensuring that AI systems support equitable and just medical practices [25].

5.2 Balancing Accuracy and Interpretability

One of the fundamental challenges in implementing explainability in GenAI systems is the trade-off between accuracy and interpretability. Generative adversarial networks (GANs) can generate realistic synthetic medical images that assist in training other AI systems, while variational autoencoders (VAEs) are capable of modeling patient data distributions for personalized treatment recommendations. However, these models often achieve their accuracy through deep neural network layers that are difficult to interpret, making it challenging for clinicians to understand the underlying logic of the AI's outputs [26].

Explainable AI (XAI) frameworks, which include methods like SHAP (SHapley Additive exPlanations) and LIME (Local Interpretable Model-agnostic Explanations), attempt to bridge this gap by providing interpretable insights without compromising too much on accuracy [27, 28].

5.3 Case Studies on Explainability in GenAI

In molecular drug optimization, generative models generate potential drug compounds. While these models accelerate drug discovery, their opaque nature can obscure the rationale behind selecting specific compounds. Improving explainability via visualization tools and interpretable model layers can assist researchers in understanding and validating AI-generated recommendations [29].

GANs are employed in medical imaging to enhance image reconstruction and segmentation. However, the complexity of these models often leads to a lack of transparency, making it difficult for clinicians to trust AI-generated images. XAI techniques, like feature attribution methods, can provide insights into how models process and generate images, fostering greater confidence in AI-assisted diagnostics [30].

6 Regulatory Frameworks for Generative AI in Healthcare

6.1 FDA Regulation of AI/ML-Based Medical Devices and HIPAA

The ***Food and Drug Administration (FDA)*** plays a pivotal role in regulating AI/ML-based medical devices in the United States. The agency has approved numerous AI/ML-enabled devices, primarily through the 510(k) clearance pathway, which emphasizes substantial equivalence to existing devices [31]. ***Health Insurance Portability and Accountability Act (HIPAA)*** governs the privacy and security of health information, ensuring that AI applications comply with data protection standards. The integration of AI in healthcare must balance innovation with patient privacy, as AI systems often require access to large datasets. HIPAA compliance is crucial for maintaining trust and protecting sensitive health information, especially as AI technologies become more prevalent in clinical settings [32].

6.2 GDPR and the AI Act

The ***General Data Protection Regulation (GDPR)*** provides a comprehensive framework for data protection in the European Union, significantly impacting AI systems. It regulates personal data processing and automated decision-making, ensuring transparency, accountability, and data minimization. GDPR mandates explicit consent for data use, which can be challenging for AI systems that require large datasets for training and operation. It also grants individuals rights such as access to their data and the ability to contest automated decisions, which are crucial for maintaining trust in AI applications.

The ***AI Act*** introduces a risk-based regulatory approach, categorizing AI systems into different risk levels and imposing stricter requirements on high-risk applications, such as those in healthcare.

6.3 Global Standards for and Frameworks

Beyond national regulations, international organizations such as the ***World Health Organization (WHO)*** and the ***International Medical Device Regulators Forum (IMDRF)*** are working to create global standards for AI in healthcare. The WHO has emphasized the need for a global framework that ensures equity, ethics, and safety in the deployment of AI in healthcare, particularly in resource-limited settings [33]. The IMDRF also plays a significant role in aligning regulatory approaches for medical devices, including those incorporating AI. It focuses on creating guidelines that address the unique challenges posed by AI technologies, such as continuous learning algorithms and real-time data processing.

The development of standardized testing and assessment guidelines, such as the ***STAGER*** checklist, is essential for evaluating the reliability of generative AI in medical contexts [34]. This checklist provides a comprehensive approach to assessing AI models, addressing key dimensions like question collection and assessment techniques, thereby enhancing research quality and reporting. Human evaluation of generative AI, particularly large language models (LLMs), is also critical for ensuring safety and effectiveness. The ***QUEST*** framework offers a structured approach to evaluating AI systems, focusing on quality, understanding, expression, safety, and trust [35]. This framework aims to enhance the reliability and applicability of AI evaluations across various healthcare applications. Despite these efforts, challenges remain in achieving global consensus on GenAI standards due to varying national priorities and regulatory environments. Table 1 provides a comparison of AI regulatory frameworks in healthcare.

6.4 Validation of Generative Models in Healthcare

Generative Adversarial Networks (GANs) are validated through the creation of synthetic datasets that closely emulate real clinical data. This can involve statistical validation methods such as Jaccard similarity and K-S tests to ensure that the synthetic data maintains similar statistical characteristics to real datasets [36]. GANs are also utilized to generate synthetic medical images, which can enhance machine learning model training by providing diverse datasets. However, challenges include the need for significant computing resources and the lack of established standards for synthetic image generation. Statistical decision-making tools are employed to validate the quality of synthetic data, ensuring it meets rigorous hypothesis testing criteria [37].

Reinforcement Learning from Human Feedback (RLHF) plays a crucial role in validating generative models in healthcare by ensuring they align with human values, potentially improving patient outcomes and safety. Safe RLHF, for instance, addresses the balance between helpfulness and harmlessness, which is critical in healthcare settings [38].

Large Language Models (LLMs) are validated through comprehensive frameworks that assess their performance in clinical contexts. This includes evaluating their ability to process and understand complex medical data using clinician annotations and systematic analysis. For instance, GPT-4 has shown superior performance in understanding clinical notes, with evaluations focusing on aspects like temporality and negation [39]. The Automated Interactive Evaluation (AIE) framework provides a dynamic platform for assessing LLMs through multi-turn doctor-patient simulations, offering a realistic validation environment [40].

Hallucination in AI is a phenomenon where a model produces data that is not grounded in the input it was provided or the underlying reality it seeks to represent.

Table 1 Comparison of AI regulatory frameworks in healthcare

Regulatory body	Key Provisions	Applicability to AI in healthcare
FDA, HIPAA	Regulates AI medical devices (510(k) clearance), enforces data privacy and security under HIPAA.	Governs AI medical devices and enforces strict data privacy, ensuring balance between innovation and patient safety.
GDPR, AI Act	Requires explicit consent, data minimization, and risk-based regulation under the AI Act.	Ensures high data privacy standards and adds risk-based regulation for high-risk applications like healthcare.
WHO, IMDRF	Focuses on ethics, equity, safety (WHO), and aligning AI medical device regulations (IMDRF).	Aims for global AI standards, focusing on equitable and safe AI applications, particularly in resource-limited settings.

In healthcare, the implications of hallucinations in AI-driven systems are particularly significant, as such errors could lead to misleading diagnostics, erroneous treatment suggestions, or fabricated insights. To address these issues, hallucination tests like the Medical Domain Hallucination Test (Med-HALT) were created by integrating multiple-choice questions and answers from medical examination tests [41].

6.5 *Responsible AI*

A survey of healthcare leaders indicates a growing interest in utilizing GenAI to improve patient experience and operational efficiency [42]. As AI technologies become more pervasive in healthcare, the concept of Responsible AI (RAI) has emerged as a framework to guide their ethical and safe use. RAI encompasses the development of AI systems that are ethical, transparent, and accountable, aiming to mitigate potential negative impacts and maximize societal benefits. In other words, we can reach RAI by establishing Explainable AI (XAI) principles (see Fig. 3). A fundamental aspect of responsible AI is stakeholder engagement. This process is essential for ensuring that AI systems align with ethical standards and societal needs. Engaging stakeholders, including users, developers, and policymakers, is essential for the effective implementation of responsible AI practices [43]. Moreover, behavioral use licensing offers a legal framework to enforce ethical guidelines, ensuring that AI technologies are utilized responsibly [44]. A collaboration between Google Cloud and Mayo Clinic exemplifies the commitment to leveraging AI in healthcare while upholding high standards of patient care and data security [45]. This partnership represents a model for how healthcare institutions can work with technology providers to integrate AI in a way that is both innovative and responsible.

AI algorithms, particularly those involving deep learning, require vast amounts of computational power. The energy required to train and run these models often

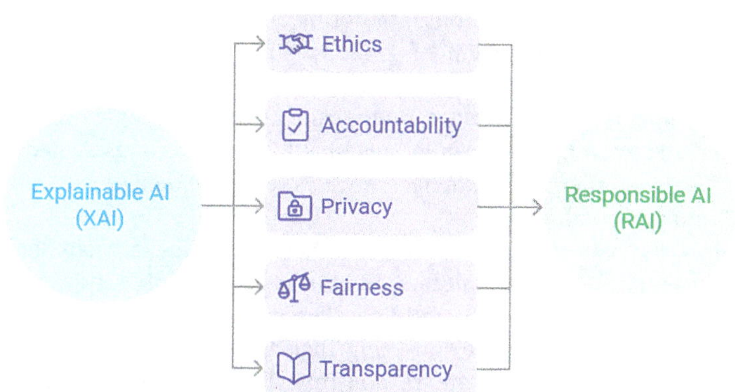

Fig. 3 Explainable AI (XAI) leads to Responsible AI (RAI)

comes from data centers that may contribute to greenhouse gas emissions. A review exploring the intersection of climate change and AI in healthcare examines these challenges, noting the need to consider the carbon footprint of AI technologies in the healthcare sector [46]. The rapid advancement and turnover of AI technologies can also lead to increased electronic waste (e-waste). As new models are developed, older systems become obsolete, contributing to the growing problem of e-waste, which can have effects on the environment if not properly disposed of or recycled. By implementing sustainable practices and developing energy-efficient AI technology, it is feasible to minimize concerns and leverage AI for the enhancement of healthcare and the environment.

7 Conclusion

The integration of generative AI (GenAI) into healthcare brings forth significant advancements. However, we cannot understate the ethical, regulatory, and technical challenges associated with these systems. GenAI's potential to transform healthcare must be tempered by its inherent risks, including algorithmic biases, issues around patient privacy, and the opacity of complex models.

The complexity of AI decision-making, especially in life-critical applications like diagnostics, necessitates clear ethical guidelines to address accountability and transparency. GenAI, while offering unprecedented capabilities in generating data, must be explainable to ensure that healthcare professionals and patients can trust and understand the decisions made. As highlighted throughout, explainability is a cornerstone in building trust in AI, especially as medical decisions increasingly rely on opaque models like generative adversarial networks (GANs) and large language models (LLMs).

Privacy concerns in GenAI are equally paramount, given the sensitive nature of medical data. While de-identification and anonymization techniques have been adopted to protect patient confidentiality, the risk of re-identification remains, underscoring the need for continuous monitoring and robust data governance frameworks. The ongoing development of global regulatory frameworks, such as the FDA's oversight of AI/ML-enabled devices and the GDPR's stringent data protection requirements, is crucial in ensuring the ethical and safe deployment of GenAI in healthcare. However, these regulations should evolve alongside technological progress to address emerging challenges, such as real-time data processing and continuous learning algorithms.

Ultimately, the path forward for GenAI in healthcare lies in balancing its transformative potential with a commitment to ethical responsibility, transparency, and patient-centered care. Continuous auditing, data diversification, and interdisciplinary collaboration will be vital to ensuring that AI not only improves healthcare outcomes but does so equitably and responsibly. The rapid pace of GenAI's adoption in healthcare must be met with equally ethical and regulatory scrutiny to safeguard both patients and healthcare professionals from unintended consequences.

References

1. Secinaro S, Calandra D, Secinaro A, Muthurangu V, Biancone P. The role of artificial intelligence in healthcare: a structured literature review. BMC Med Inform Decis Mak. 2021;21:1–23. https://doi.org/10.1186/s12911-021-01488-9.
2. Floridi L, Cowls J, Beltrametti M, Chatila R, Chazerand P, Dignum V, et al. AI4People—an ethical framework for a good AI society: opportunities, risks, principles, and recommendations. Mind Mach. 2018;28:689–707. https://doi.org/10.1007/s11023-018-9482-5.
3. Obermeyer Z, Powers B, Vogeli C, Mullainathan S. Dissecting racial bias in an algorithm used to manage the health of populations. Science. 2019;366(6464):447–53. https://doi.org/10.1126/science.aax2342.
4. Okonji OR, Yunusov K, Gordon B. Applications of Generative AI in Healthcare: algorithmic, ethical, legal and societal considerations. TechRxiv. 2024; https://doi.org/10.36227/techrxiv.171527587.75649430/v1.
5. Morley J, Floridi L, Kinsey L, Elhalal A. From what to how: an initial review of publicly available AI ethics tools, methods and research to translate principles into practices. Sci Eng Ethics. 2020;26(4):2141–68. https://doi.org/10.1007/s11948-019-00165-5.
6. Amedior NC. Ethical implications of artificial intelligence in the healthcare sector. Adv Multidiscip Sci Res J Publ. 2023;36:1–12. https://doi.org/10.22624/AIMS/ACCRABESPOKE2023P1.
7. Lawton T, Morgan P, Porter Z, Hickey S, Cunningham A, Hughes N, Iacovides I, Jia Y, Sharma V, Habli I. Clinicians risk becoming 'liability sinks' for artificial intelligence. Future healthc J. 2024;11(1):100007. https://doi.org/10.1016/j.fhj.2024.100007.
8. Anyanwu EC, Okongwu CC, Olorunsogo TO, Ayo-Farai O, Osasona F, Daraojimba OD. Artificial intelligence in healthcare: a review of ethical dilemmas and practical applications. Int Med Sci Res J. 2024;4(2):126–40. https://doi.org/10.51594/imsrj.v4i2.755.
9. Amann J, Blasimme A, Vayena E, Frey D, Madai VI, Precise4Q Consortium. Explainability for artificial intelligence in healthcare: a multidisciplinary perspective. BMC Med Inform Decis Mak. 2020;20:1–9. https://doi.org/10.1186/s12911-020-01332-6.
10. Rajpurkar P, Irvin J, Zhu K, Yang B, Mehta H, Duan T, et al. CheXNet: Radiologist-Level Pneumonia Detection on Chest X-Rays with Deep Learning. ArXiv:171105225 [Cs, Stat]. 2017. https://arxiv.org/abs/1711.05225v3.
11. Mohammad Amini M, Jesus M, Fanaei Sheikholeslami D, Alves P, Hassanzadeh Benam A, Hariri F. Artificial intelligence ethics and challenges in healthcare applications: a comprehensive review in the context of the European GDPR mandate. Mach Learn Knowl Extr. 2023;5(3):1023–35. https://doi.org/10.3390/make5030053.
12. Biswas A, Talukdar W. Intelligent clinical documentation: harnessing generative AI for patient-centric clinical note generation. Int J Innov Sci Res Technol. 2024:994–1008. https://doi.org/10.38124/ijisrt/ijisrt24may1483. https://arxiv.org/abs/2405.18346v1
13. Chen Y, Esmaeilzadeh P. Generative AI in medical practice: in-depth exploration of privacy and security challenges. J Med Internet Res. 2024;26:e53008. https://doi.org/10.2196/53008.
14. Kushida CA, Nichols DA, Jadrnicek R, Miller R, Walsh JK, Griffin K. Strategies for de-identification and anonymization of electronic health record data for use in multicenter research studies. Med Care. 2012;50 Suppl(Suppl):S82–S101. https://doi.org/10.1097/MLR.0b013e3182585355.
15. Rocher L, Hendrickx JM, de Montjoye YA. Estimating the success of re-identifications in incomplete datasets using generative models. Nat Commun. 2019;10(1):3069. https://doi.org/10.1038/s41467-019-10933-3.
16. Goodfellow IJ, Shlens J, Szegedy C. Explaining and harnessing adversarial examples. ArXiv:1412.6572 [Cs, Stat]. 2015. https://arxiv.org/abs/1412.6572v3
17. Wang Y, Liu C, Zhou K, Zhu T, Han X. Towards regulatory generative AI in ophthalmology healthcare: a security and privacy perspective. Br J Ophthalmol, bjo-2024-325167. 2024. Advance online publication. https://doi.org/10.1136/bjo-2024-325167.

18. Mehrabi N, Morstatter F, Saxena N, Lerman K, Galstyan A. A survey on bias and fairness in machine learning. ACM Comput Surv (CSUR). 2021;54(6):1–35. https://doi.org/10.1145/3457607.
19. Challen R, Denny J, Pitt M, Gompels L, Edwards T, Tsaneva-Atanasova K. Artificial intelligence, bias and clinical safety. BMJ Qual Saf. 2019;28(3):231–7. https://doi.org/10.1136/bmjqs-2018-008370.
20. Ferrara E. Fairness and bias in artificial intelligence: a brief survey of sources, impacts, and mitigation strategies. Sci. 2023;6(1):3. https://doi.org/10.3390/sci6010003.
21. Templin T, Perez MW, Sylvia S, Leek J, Sinnott-Armstrong N. Addressing 6 challenges in generative AI for digital health: a scoping review. PLOS Digit Health. 2024;3(5):e0000503. https://doi.org/10.1371/journal.pdig.0000503.
22. Olmos CL, Neophytou A, Sengupta S, Papadopoulos DP. Latent Directions: A Simple Pathway to Bias Mitigation in Generative AI. ArXiv:2406.06352. 2024. https://arxiv.org/abs/2406.06352
23. Adamson AS, Smith A. Machine learning and health care disparities in dermatology. JAMA Dermatol. 2018;154(11):1247–8. https://doi.org/10.1001/jamadermatol.2018.2348.
24. Schneider J. Explainable Generative AI (GenXAI): a survey, conceptualization, and research agenda. Artif Intell Rev. 2024;57(11):289. https://doi.org/10.1007/s10462-024-10916-x.
25. Sai S, Gaur A, Sai R, Chamola V, Guizani M, Rodrigues JJ. Generative AI for transformative healthcare: a comprehensive study of emerging models, applications, case studies and limitations. IEEE Access. 2024. https://doi.org/10.1109/ACCESS.2024.3367715.
26. Rudin C. Stop explaining black box machine learning models for high stakes decisions and use interpretable models instead. Nat Mach Intell. 2019;1(5):206–15. https://doi.org/10.1038/s42256-019-0048-x.
27. Lundberg, S, Lee, SI. A Unified Approach to Interpreting Model Predictions. In Advances in Neural Information Processing Systems. 2017;30. https://arxiv.org/abs/1705.07874.
28. Ribeiro MT, Singh S, Guestrin C. "Why should I trust you?" Explaining the predictions of any classifier. In: Proceedings of the 22nd ACM SIGKDD international conference on knowledge discovery and data mining. 2016. pp. 1135–44. https://doi.org/10.1145/2939672.2939778.
29. Ijiga AC, Peace AE, Idoko IP, Agbo DO, Harry KD, Ezebuka CI, Ukatu IE. Ethical considerations in implementing generative AI for healthcare supply chain optimization: a cross-country analysis across India, the United Kingdom, and the United States of America. Int J Biol Pharma Sci Arch. 2024;7(01):048–63. https://doi.org/10.53771/ijbpsa.2024.7.1.0015.
30. Musalamadugu TS, Kannan H. Generative AI for medical imaging analysis and applications. Future Med AI. 2023;1(2). doi: https://doi.org/10.2217/fmai-2023-0004.
31. Joshi G, Jain A, Araveeti SR, Adhikari S, Garg H, Bhandari M. FDA-approved artificial intelligence and machine learning (AI/ML)-enabled medical devices: an updated landscape. Electronics. 2024;13(3):498. https://doi.org/10.3390/electronics13030498.
32. Jadon A, Kumar S. Leveraging generative AI models for synthetic data generation in healthcare: balancing research and privacy. In: 2023 international conference on smart applications, communications and networking (SmartNets). IEEE; 2023. p. 1–4. https://doi.org/10.1109/SmartNets58706.2023.10215825.
33. WHO. Ethics and governance of artificial intelligence for health: WHO guidance. 2021. Available at: https://www.who.int/publications/i/item/9789240029200
34. Chen J, Zhu L, Mou W, Lin A, Zeng D, Qi C, et al. STAGER checklist: standardized testing and assessment guidelines for evaluating generative artificial intelligence reliability. iMetaOmics. 2024;1(1):e7. https://doi.org/10.1002/imo2.7.
35. Thomas T, Sivarajkumar S, Kapoor S, Stolyar AV, Polanska K, McCarthy KR, Osterhoudt H, Wu X, Visweswaran S, Fu S, Mathur P, Cacciamani GE, Sun C, Peng Y, Wang Y. A literature review and framework for human evaluation of generative large language models in healthcare. 2024. ArXiv.org. https://arxiv.org/abs/2405.02559v1

36. Arvanitis TN, White S, Harrison S, Chaplin R, Despotou G. A method for machine learning generation of realistic synthetic datasets for validating healthcare applications. Health Informatics J. 2022;28(2):14604582221077000. https://doi.org/10.1177/14604582221077000.
37. Gonzalez-Abril L, Angulo C, Ortega JA, Lopez-Guerra JL. Statistical validation of synthetic data for lung cancer patients generated by using generative adversarial networks. Electronics. 2022;11(20):3277. https://doi.org/10.3390/electronics11203277.
38. Dai J, Pan X, Sun R, Ji J, Xu X, Liu M, Wang Y, Yang Y. Safe RLHF: Safe reinforcement learning from human feedback. ArXiv:2310.12773. 2023. https://arxiv.org/abs/2310.12773
39. Liu D, Ding C, Bold D, Bouvier M, Lu J, Shickel B, Jabaley CS, Zhang W, Park S, Young MJ, Wainwright MS. Evaluation of General Large Language Models in Contextually Assessing Semantic Concepts Extracted from Adult Critical Care Electronic Health Record Notes. ArXiv:2401.13588. 2024. https://arxiv.org/abs/2401.13588v1
40. Liao Y, Meng Y, Wang Y, Liu H, Wang Y, Wang Y. Automatic Interactive Evaluation for Large Language Models with State Aware Patient Simulator. ArXiv:2403.08495. 2024. https://arxiv.org/abs/2403.08495v4
41. Pal A, Umapathi LK, Sankarasubbu M. Med-halt: Medical domain hallucination test for large language models. ArXiv:2307.15343. 2023. https://arxiv.org/abs/2307.15343v2
42. Generative AI in healthcare: adoption trends and what's next. McKinsey & Company. Retrieved 28 July 2024, from https://www.mckinsey.com/industries/healthcare/our-insights/generative-ai-in-healthcare-adoption-trends-and-whats-next
43. Deshpande A, Sharp H. Responsible AI systems: who are the stakeholders? In: Proceedings of the 2022 AAAI/ACM conference on AI, ethics, and society; 2022. p. 227–36. https://doi.org/10.1145/3514094.3534187.
44. Contractor D, McDuff D, Haines JK, Lee J, Hines C, Hecht B, et al. Behavioral use licensing for responsible AI. In: Proceedings of the 2022 ACM conference on fairness, accountability, and transparency; 2022. p. 778–88. https://doi.org/10.1145/3531146.3533143.
45. The Lancet Regional Health-Europe. Embracing generative AI in health care. Lancet Reg Health Eur. 2023;30:100677. https://doi.org/10.1016/j.lanepe.2023.100677.
46. Ueda D, Walston SL, Fujita S, Fushimi Y, Tsuboyama T, Kamagata K, Yamada A, Yanagawa M, Ito R, Fujima N, Kawamura M, Nakaura T, Matsui Y, Tatsugami F, Fujioka T, Nozaki T, Hirata K, Naganawa S. Climate change and artificial intelligence in healthcare: review and recommendations towards a sustainable future. Diagn Interv Imaging. 2024;S2211-5684(24):00138–4. https://doi.org/10.1016/j.diii.2024.06.002. Advance online publication.

www.ingramcontent.com/pod-product-compliance
Lightning Source LLC
Chambersburg PA
CBHW071436090325
23216CB00001B/16
9783031829628